THE NUTRITIONAL HANDGUIDE

**50 Research-Backed Health Tips
Your Go-To Wellness Guide
To Healthy Aging**

J.E. MILLER

Health Books USA

Copyright © 2025 By J.E. Miller

All rights reserved. No part of this book may be reproduced, stored in a retrieval system, or transmitted in any form or by any means, electronic, mechanical, photocopying, recording, or otherwise, without the prior written permission of the author and publisher except in the case of written quotations in articles or reviews.

Disclaimer: The contents of this book are for informational purposes only and are not intended to serve as a substitute for professional medical advice to treat, diagnose, or cure any health problem. Therefore, the author and publisher are not responsible or liable to any person or entity for any loss, damage, injury caused directly or indirectly by applying the information found in this book. Always consult with your doctor before following any health advice.

ISBN Hardcover: 979-8-9867024-3-8
ISBN Paperback: 979-8-9867024-4-5
ISBN eBook: 979-8-9867024-5-2

Library of Congress Control Number: 2025921100

Cover art work and formatting by 100covers.com

Contents

Introduction

Tip 1 - Antioxidants: Winning the Daily Anti-Aging Battle Against Free Radicals and Oxidative Stress	1
Tip 2 - Raw Juices: A Health Insurance Policy	8
Tip 3 - Organic Apple Cider Vinegar Remedy	14
Tip 4 - Alcohol Health Benefits?	18
Tip 5 - Healthier Cocktails	22
Tip 6 - Red Wine's Potential Health Benefits	25
Tip 7 - Beer vs. Wine	30
Tip 8 - Health Concerns with Drinking Alcohol on an Empty Stomach	33
Tip 9 - Potential Problems with Drinking Beer (or Anything) Out of Aluminum Cans	36
Tip 10 - Hangover Prevention and Recovery Remedies	39
Tip 11 - Milk "Liver Helper" Thistle	43
Tip 12 - Heartburn Remedy	46
Tip 13 - Naturally Getting "The Red Out"	49
Tip 14 - Overcoming Baggy Dark Circles	52

Tip 15 - Naturally Relieving Coughs and Cottonmouth	59
Tip 16 - Apples Keep the Lung Doctor Away	61
Tip 17 - Fruits and Vegetables for Smokers and Ex-Smokers	64
Tip 18 - Vitamins for Smokers and Ex-Smokers	67
Tip 19 - The Antioxidant Powers of Grape Seed "Youth" Extract	72
Tip 20 - Hot Peppers Healthy Buzz	78
Tip 21 - Sweet Potatoes: A Perfect Munchie Food	81
Tip 22 - Garlic and Your Health	85
Tip 23 - What's the Deal with Red and Processed Meat?	88
Tip 24 - Beating Table Salt's Deadly Addiction	94
Tip 25 - Overcoming Sugar Addiction	99
Tip 26 - Kicking the Artificial Sweeteners Non-Nutritive Habit	104
Tip 27 - Hold the Canola Oil	108
Tip 28 - Soy Health Alert	111
Tip 29 - Celery Health	115
Tip 30 - Importance of Vitamin B Complex	117
Tip 31 - Health Benefits of Raw Nuts and Seeds	121
Tip 32 - Scoring the Best Bread	126
Tip 33 - Wheatgrass Juice "Healing" Shots	131
Tip 34 - Organic Produce or Bust?	134
Tip 35 - Cruciferous Vegetables for Cancer Prevention and Overall Better Health	140
Tip 36 - Lemon Aid	145
Tip 37 - Tea Break	149
Tip 38 - Coffee's Wake Up Concerns	155
Tip 39 - Melatonin Nightcap	158
Tip 40 - Your Tongue is a Window Into Your Health	162

Tip 41 - Beating Gout	164
Tip 42 - A Daily Parasite Protection Plan	167
Tip 43 - Controlling Stress	172
Tip 44 - Preventing and Reversing Gray Hairs	175
Tip 45 - Resistance (Isometric) Exercises: A 20 Minute Workout and Detox Routine	180
Tip 46 - Why We Need Sunshine (Vitamin D)	188
Tip 47 - Brewer's Yeast: A Complete Meal	193
Tip 48 - Berries Are Brain Food	196
Tip 49 - Omega Fatty Acids Build and Maintain a Healthy Brain	198
Tip 50 - Brain Cells Regrow After All	205
References	211

Introduction

The Nutritional Handguide contains 50 health tips geared to improve your overall health regardless of your lifestyle. Though it's no surprise that a poor diet is the primary cause of most health problems. And "The risk that poor diets pose to mortality and morbidity is now greater than the combined risks of unsafe sex, alcohol, drug and tobacco use," according to a report by the Global Panel on Agriculture and Food Systems for Nutrition. It's also linked to one in five premature deaths caused by diabetes, cardiovascular diseases, and cancer.

The daily challenge to achieving a healthier diet, of course, is the craving for processed foods that research finds can be as addictive as cocaine or heroin. These foods, which are normally high in addictive salt, sugar, or saturated fats, are designed to maximize food companies' profits, but they also maximize your risks of chronic diseases. Nevertheless, research finds that half of US adults have a chronic disease caused by a poor diet or unhealthy eating habits.

The philosopher and teacher Socrates (469-399 BCE) put healthy eating in perspective when he stated: "Thou shouldst eat to live; not live to eat." And, therefore, you are what you eat (and drink).

Healthy Food Is Medicine

Since the beginning of civilization, humans have relied on whole (unprocessed) foods as nourishment or medicine. As Hippocrates (460-370 BCE), the father of modern medicine proclaimed: "Let thy food be thy medicine and thy medicine be thy food." The good news is that this timeless advice also applies to partying—there are healthy ways to help counteract it.

For example, "smokers and high alcohol consumers" who also consumed foods high in flavonoids (antioxidants) such as apples, oranges, pears, blueberries, broccoli, and green tea reduced their risk of "all-cause, cardiovascular and cancer-related mortality [death]," according to the study, Flavonoid Intake is Associated with Lower Mortality in the Danish Diet Cancer and Health Cohort. Analyzing data from diets of 56,048 Danes over 23 years, researchers found those with the lowest risk of cardiovascular disease-related mortality consumed around 500 mg of flavonoids a day, which equals approximately a half cup of blueberries, a half cup of broccoli, and a cup of green tea. But the "threshold was higher, approximately 1000 mg/d for cancer-related mortality." And "The strongest associations observed between flavonoids and mortality was in smokers and high alcohol consumers, with higher intakes being more beneficial."

Furthermore, according to the study, Higher Diet Quality Relates to Decelerated Epigenetic [Biological] Aging, researchers "analyzed data from 1,995 participants (mean age, 67 years; 55% women) of the Framingham Heart Study Offspring Cohort...[and found] that better diet quality was associated with decelerated biological aging, providing a promising avenue to explore the beneficial effects of diet on prolonged lifespans. This effect seems to be more prominent for those who have a history of smoking." So a healthy diet seems to be the real fountain of youth for all.

Plus, "Light and moderate alcohol intake might have a protective effect on all-cause and CVD-specific mortality in US adults," according to the study, Relationship of Alcohol Consumption to All-Cause, Cardiovascular, and Cancer-Related Mortality in US Adults, which included 333,247 participants.

The 50 Health Tips

My background is a lifelong passion for nutrition. The following 50 health tips cover over 30 years of health research and include hundreds of research studies to ensure you receive some of the best nutritional advice available. They also focus on a holistic approach, which treats the body as a whole to improve your overall health, as taught by Hippocrates.

But step one to staying healthy is learning how to become a health expert, which is the underlying goal of the book. It helps put you in control of your health, and it's not hard to accomplish.

J.E. Miller
Health Researcher

The 50 Health Tips

Tip 1

Antioxidants: Winning the Daily Anti-Aging Battle Against Free Radicals and Oxidative Stress

We're all under daily attack from free radicals that, if left unchecked, can cause oxidative stress, an all too often condition that's linked to everything from premature aging to chronic disease.

A free radical is created when one of your atoms loses an electron in its valance shell or outermost orbital, which is required to maintain its stability. Pairing electrons achieve stability. But once unpaired, the free radical is not only unstable but also highly reactive as it now searches for an electron to regain its stability. In its quest, it can steal one from any atom or molecule (group of atoms) it encounters, thus turning it into a free radical. And without antioxidant help, it becomes a dangerous chain reaction or domino effect called oxidative stress, which harms cells.

Free radicals are mainly known as reactive oxygen species (ROS) and reactive nitrogen species (RNS) that are created from internal (endogenous) and exterior (exogenous) sources. Exterior sources of free radicals include air pollution, radiation (e.g., nuclear power plants, x-rays, microwaves, cell phone towers, mobile phones, 5G), stress, cigarette smoke, alcohol, pharmaceutical drugs, chemicals, pesticides, fried foods, sodium nitrite, table salt, table sugar, white rice, and trans fats.

Internal sources of free radicals are mainly created, however, as a normal byproduct of breathing oxygen, metabolizing food, and immune system functions—some even fight off pathogens and are needed for cell signaling. So free radicals are a double-edged sword: some are beneficial—but too many are harmful.

The health problems begin when you have more free radicals in circulation than antioxidants (stable molecules that keep them in check). Even though most free radicals have a very short life span (around a millionth of a second), an overabundance can trigger oxidative stress, also known as a free radical and antioxidant imbalance that alters proper cell functions and can even cause premature cell death by damaging its membrane lipids (fats), proteins, mitochondria, DNA, and RNA, which numerous studies have linked to causing premature aging (wrinkles), arthritis, atherosclerosis, hypertension, cardiovascular diseases, respiratory diseases, eye diseases, autoimmune disorders, diabetes, osteoporosis, multiple sclerosis, Parkinson's disease, Alzheimer's disease, and cancer—you name it.

Though the damaging consequences of unchecked free radicals and oxidative stress are usually first seen on someone's face. An extreme example of this is the before and after pictures of a crystal methamphetamine (meth) addict, who is usually severely deficient in antioxidants by not eating right. In a few years, for instance, a twenty-year-old male looks years older: the meth's free radicals significantly sped up his aging process by causing severe oxidative stress damage to his skin's collagen and elastin connective tissues.

Other signs of oxidative stress include hair, hearing, vision, and memory loss.

A Brief History: Free Radicals and Aging

In 1900, Moses Gomberg, Professor of Chemistry at the University of Michigan, first speculated on the existence of organic free radicals. And in 1954, Dr. Rebeca Gershman and Dr. Daniel Gilbert proposed the free radical theory of oxygen toxicity or how oxygen (ROS) causes free radicals. Then, in 1956, Dr. Denham Harman first proposed the free radical theory of aging with his article, Aging: A Theory Based on Free Radical and Radiation Chemistry. According to Dr. Harman, free radicals are highly unstable and reactive chemical subspecies that can tear apart the molecules required for life's normal processes, including a cell's mitochondria, the cellular powerhouses that create energy for your body and help determine one's life span.

In his 1992 follow-up review, the Free Radical Theory of Aging, Dr. Harman finds that, "The data supporting this theory indicate that average life expectancy at birth may be increased by five or more years, by nutritious low caloric diets supplemented with one or more free radical reaction inhibitors [antioxidants]."

Their research, along with other scientists, would eventually help make the word "antioxidant" a household name.

Your Antioxidant Defenses

Antioxidants act as free radical scavengers and electron donors—they not only search out and neutralize or destroy free radicals, ending the electron stealing, but also provide an electron to re-stabilize the attacked atom or molecule. They also prevent free radicals from being formed in the first place. The goal is to maintain a healthy balance of antioxidants (internal and external) to defend against an overabundance of them.

Fortunately, your cells contain multiple internal antioxidant defenses that guard against free radicals and oxidative stress generated by normal bodily functions and external sources. These powerful antioxidants include glutathione (a.k.a. the master antioxidant for its versatility), superoxide dismutase, catalase, coenzyme Q10, and alpha lipoic acid. For instance, cancer and Alzheimer's disease patients have lower levels of these cell-protecting antioxidants. Researchers from Baylor College of Medicine in Houston also found that adults hospitalized with Covid-19 had a severe glutathione deficiency resulting in oxidative stress damage.

On the other hand, the best sources of external antioxidants include over 8,000 plant polyphenols (plant defense compounds that contain powerful antioxidants) also known as flavonoids (e.g., catechins, anthocyanins, proanthocyanidins, kaempferol, quercetin) and phenolic acids (e.g., ferulic acid, caffeic acid, p-coumaric acid, ellagic acid, gallic acid) that are found in whole grains, fruits, vegetables, nuts, seeds, and tea. And over 600 plant carotenoids (plant pigment defense compounds that contain powerful antioxidants) including alpha-carotene, beta-carotene, lycopene, lutein, and zeaxanthin that are found in fruits, vegetables, nuts, seeds, herbs, teas, and red wine. Plus, there's the powerful carotenoid antioxidant astaxanthin that gives salmon, red trout, red snapper, krill, lobster, crayfish, crabs, and shrimp their red-pinkish color. Red yeast is another good source.

Vitamin A, vitamin B2 (riboflavin), vitamin C, vitamin D, vitamin E, and the minerals selenium, copper, and zinc also act as powerful external antioxidants. They are found in various fruits, vegetables, meats, seafood, whole grains, beans, nuts, and seeds.

Most antioxidants are either water-soluble or fat-soluble. Water-soluble antioxidants (e.g., glutathione, catalase, and vitamin C) protect bodily fluids inside and outside of cells while fat-soluble antioxidants (e.g., vitamin A, vitamin E, and coenzyme Q10) protect cellular lipids (membranes).

Antioxidant Diet

Here's how to get the variety of antioxidants needed to guard against free radicals and oxidative stress:

- Consume five to seven antioxidant-rich fruits and vegetables a day. Usually the more colorful the produce, the more plant antioxidants. And when possible, purchase organic produce. Research finds they contain more antioxidants than non-organic or conventionally grown produce (see Tip 34 - Organic Produce or Bust?).

- Consume antioxidant-rich beans such as red beans, red kidney beans, pinto beans, and black beans. (A 2004 USDA study on the top food sources of antioxidants surprisingly found that small red beans to contain the most antioxidants, followed by wild blueberries, red kidney beans, and pinto beans.)

- Consume antioxidant-rich raw nuts and seeds. For example, a mixture of almonds, walnuts, pecans, cashews, Brazil nuts, sunflower seeds, and pumpkin seeds (see Tip 31 - Health Benefits of Raw Nuts and Seeds).

- Consume antioxidant-rich whole grains such as whole wheat bread, whole oats, whole barley, and brown rice. Whole grains mean they still contain their bran, germ, and endosperm (see Tip 32 - Scoring the Best Bread).

- Consume antioxidant-rich spices such as turmeric, oregano, basil, thyme, rosemary, saffron, ginger, black pepper, and cayenne pepper.

- Consume foods that are sources of glutathione, superoxide dismutase, catalase, coenzyme Q10, and alpha lipoic acid, such as broccoli, cabbage, cauliflower, kale, garlic, spinach, sweet potatoes, avocados, and Brewer's yeast.

- Consume antioxidant-rich wild salmon, red trout, red snapper, lobster, crayfish, crabs, and shrimp.

- Drink tea. All teas contain potent antioxidants that help detoxify your body of harmful free radicals (see Tip 37 - Tea Break).

- Take antioxidant supplements. It's best to get your antioxidants mainly from your diet; otherwise, take around 100 mg of vitamin C, and 200 IU of vitamin E mixed tocopherols. Then in the afternoon, take a 200 mg grape seed extract supplement (see Tip 19 - Antioxidant Powers of Grape Seed "Youth" Extract). These antioxidants also help to rejuvenate your cell's antioxidant defenses.

How Are Your Antioxidant Levels?

Remember that the longer your antioxidant levels remain low, your potential risks of premature aging and chronic disease remain high. If you are curious, a free radical or oxidative stress test is available at some medical clinics and over-the-counter.

At any rate, if you are consuming enough plant antioxidants and avoiding most junk foods and other toxins, your free radical levels should be under control. Premature aging is a big clue.

Winning the daily battle against free radicals and oxidative stress is the first step to maintain a youthful mind and body. And the first step to counteract overindulging.

Tip 2

Raw Juices: A Health Insurance Policy

Raw fruits and vegetables are essential sources of plant protein (amino acids), vitamins, minerals, antioxidants, and enzymes needed to nourish your estimated 37 trillion cells while guarding them from disease. So getting your daily servings is one of the most important health goals anyone can ever accomplish.

How many servings do you consume a day? The US recommended daily allowance (RDA) is five a day or two fruits and three vegetables. Although a meta-analysis study (multiple scientific studies) from the Norwegian University of Science and Technology and the Imperial College London, found "for coronary heart disease, stroke, cardiovascular disease and all-cause mortality the lowest risk was observed at 800 g/day (10 servings/day)." They found it could save approximately 7.8 million premature deaths worldwide. Therefore, whoever consumes the most fruits and vegetables potentially lives the healthiest and the longest.

Juicing: Unlocking Nutrients

A quick way to get your daily servings of raw fruits and vegetables (that only 10% of Americans attain) is to juice them for it takes more than a few pounds of produce to make a 10-ounce drink. Otherwise, it would take a cow or a horse to chew them all down!

This makes raw fruit and vegetable juices a concentrated source of plant protein, vitamins, minerals, antioxidants, and enzymes.

Here's how juicing works: when you push produce through a vegetable juicer, it instantly unlocks the nutrients sealed inside their cell walls. Now your body can quickly assimilate them and reap their rewards instead of waiting for your digestive system to complete this job. So in a sense, raw juices are pre-digested.

For instance, eating a carrot whole can take hours to digest completely, and you may not absorb all of its nutrients unless you chew it well. But when you juice a carrot, it breaks down and removes the plant's cell walls (cellulose), allowing for the majority of its nutrients to be quickly absorbed into your bloodstream, which then delivers them to where they are needed. This includes carrot's substantial source of beta-carotene and alpha-carotene, which your body converts to vitamin A, required for a healthy immune system, skin, and vision.

Raw Juicing Health Benefits

Studies find that consuming raw fruit and vegetable juices helps prevent premature aging, cardiovascular diseases, and all-cause mortality.

They also find that raw produce provides more nutrients for improving mental health than cooked or canned produce. Plus, raw juices' concentrated source of antioxidants help prevent the "chronic accumulation of reactive oxygen species [ROS free radicals] in the brain may exhaust antioxidant capacity, including antioxidant vitamins, and lead to the onset and progression of Alzheimer's disease," according to the study, Fruit and Vegetable Juices and Alzheimer's Disease [AD]: The Kame Project, which included 1,836 Japanese Americans. Researchers found that drinking juices high in polyphenols (antioxidants) at least three times per week "was associated with a substantially decreased risk of Alzheimer's disease."

Juicing is also a remedy for maintaining a healthy weight, according to the study, Health Benefit of Vegetable/Fruit Juice-Based Diet: Role of Microbiome. Researchers found that a vegetable and fruit juice-based diet positively affects the microbiome—your gut's estimated 100 trillion microbes (mainly bacteria) and their genomes—by decreasing gut Firmicutes bacteria associated with increased weight gain while increasing gut Bacteroidetes bacteria associated with decreased weight gain. (Note: The terms "microbiome" and "microbiota" are often used interchangeably, but there is a distinction. The microbiome refers to the microorganisms and their genes found in a specific environment, such as the gut, mouth, lungs, vagina, or skin. And the microbiota refers to just the microorganisms, such as bacteria, viruses, and fungi found in that environment.)

Importance of Raw (Alive) Produce

Since your cells are alive, obviously, they thrive better on a diet of more alive or raw produce than on more dead or overcooked foods. They are alive because their life-giving enzymes are still intact; temperatures over 117 degrees F destroys them.

Enzymes, the catalysis (spark plugs) of life, are proteins that create hundreds of chemical reactions required to keep you alive, healthy, and youthful. They're also vital for healthy digestion and energy production.

So for healthier cells, make sure to consume raw produce with each meal.

Juicing Options

The juicing options are either to purchase a juice drink at a health food store or juice bar for anywhere from $5 to $10 or buy a juicer and juice at home. After the cost of a juicer, the produce to make a juice will cost around $3, or the price of a good beer on happy hour.

The cost of a decent juicer ranges between $70 to $150, although high-end juicers start around $300. There are two main types of juicers: the original high-speed centrifugal juicer and the newer slow-speed cold press juicer. Many now, however, prefer cold press juicers because the high-speed (heat generated) centrifugal juicers can destroy some enzymes, vitamins, and minerals.

Either way, consuming raw fresh juice is always a better option than drinking bottled or canned juices for they must be heated to pasteurization (162 degrees F) to prevent the growth of pathogens, which besides destroying the plant's enzymes, also reduces their levels of vitamins, minerals, and antioxidants.

What's Best to Juice?

For years, carrots have been the main vegetable of many juices because they give it substance, a sweet taste, and some potent nutrients. Nevertheless, all produce is healthy, so take your pick. Think variety, the spice of life.

But whenever possible, mainly juice organic produce to avoid drinking a cocktail of pesticides since most conventional produce contains more than one pesticide (see Tip 35 - Organic Produce or Bust?). Though whether you juice organic or conventional produce, make sure to wash them well to remove any harmful bacteria. And to prevent wasting valuable juice, push produce slowly through the juicer to give it enough time to break down or release the plant's nutrients.

Here's an ultimate raw juice example (a V10): three organic carrots, two organic celery stalks, organic lettuce leave, half of organic tomato, half of medium beet, broccoli flower, onion slice, garlic clove, small sweet potato, and an organic apple.

And since juices taste better cold, juice into a cold mug or add an ice cube.

How to Consume a Raw Juice

After juicing, it's important to drink your juice immediately because it can lose nutrients in a short time due to oxidation, the free radical effect of exposure to oxygen. But drink slowly. Raw juices are very concentrated. Guzzling one down could cause indigestion or bloating, as with other beverages. Remember that the digestive process starts with your saliva enzymes. So first mix the juice around in your mouth before slowly swallowing.

And since there are a lot of natural sugars in any juice, eat something healthy to control sugar (glucose) levels. For instance, a hardboiled egg or a slice of fish, which also makes for an ideal meal.

Juicing and Your Fiber Needs

It's also important to consume vegetables "whole" because juicing removes their insoluble fiber (your intestinal broom), which absorbs water and thereby gives your colon its required roughage and bulk needed to prevent constipation. There is, however, soluble fiber in raw juices, which dissolves in water and forms a gel that helps you absorb more nutrients while removing bad LDL cholesterol and saturated fats from circulation. Soluble fiber is also vital food (prebiotics) for your beneficial gut bacteria (microbes).

Although only 5% of Americans reach the RDA of 25 to 30 grams of fiber (soluble and insoluble). To ensure you do, daily consume a mixed vegetable salad and some whole grains, beans, nuts, and seeds.

Juicing Motivation

Once you get the hang of juicing, it should only take around 10 minutes to wash the produce, juice them, and then clean the juicer. Time well spent—juicing is like taking out a long-term health insurance policy. Plus, your digestive system needs a break sometimes too.

Try to drink a glass of fresh raw juice at least three times a week.

Tip 3

Organic Apple Cider Vinegar Remedy

A perfect drink to start your day with is to mix a tablespoon of organic apple cider vinegar in spring water. It helps revitalize your trillions of cells while guarding them against disease. Reportedly prescribed by Hippocrates in 400 BCE, it's about as close as you can get to the fountain of health in a tablespoon.

Overall, organic apple cider vinegar is a remedy to overcome fatigue, depression, lung congestion, colds, sore throats, ear infections, food poisoning, indigestion, inflammation, high LDL cholesterol, high blood sugar, and heartburn. Research also finds that it reduces body weight (fat). To lose weight, for instance, consume a tablespoon with each meal.

There's no need to read any research studies to prove its worth. Just give it a try for a few weeks.

A Potent Blend of Organic Nutrients

A tablespoon of organic apple cider vinegar contains B vitamins, vitamin C, potassium, calcium, magnesium, manganese, sodium, phosphorus, and flavonoid antioxidants that also increase your levels of the antioxidants glutathione, superoxide dismutase, catalase, and vitamin E. And it's a good source of enzymes, keys to vitality and healthy digestion.

Organic apple cider vinegar also contains soluble fiber (prebiotics) and beneficial live bacteria (probiotics) needed to build and maintain a healthy gut microbiota, your gut's trillions of microbes (bacteria). A healthy gut microbiota, for instance, is essential for proper digestion, vitamin production, and immune functions by protecting against the colonization of harmful microorganisms. It makes up around 70% of your immune system.

And researchers find "for the first time that the bacterial microbiota for the industrial production of organic apple cider vinegar is clearly more heterogeneous [diverse] than the bacterial microbiota for the industrial production of conventional apple cider vinegar," according to the study, Comparison of Cultivable Acetic Acid Bacterial Microbiota in Organic and Conventional Apple Cider Vinegar.

Organic apple cider vinegar also contains acetic acid and malic acid, which contain antimicrobial, antibacterial, antifungal, antiviral, and antiparasitic properties. These acids help cleanse your body of disease-causing bugs while helping to lose weight.

Cold Prevention and Relief

The saying, "An apple a day keeps the doctor away," should also apply to drinking a tablespoon of organic apple cider vinegar a day for it also helps to keep you well. I started drinking it daily in 1998 to help guard against catching a cold and (knocking on wood) I've had only four colds since. Many others have seen similar results.

Here's how to use it to guard against colds: on rising, drink a tablespoon of organic apple cider vinegar in spring water. Then anytime you feel like you're catching a cold (or encounter someone who has a cold), drink another tablespoon as soon as possible (though you may need to drink more until feeling better). This is a crucial step to recall for its antimicrobial, antiviral, and other properties can eliminate many bugs before they can take hold and cause a cold. Also gargling with it quickly relieves a sore throat.

Indigestion-Upset Stomach Prevention and Relief

How's your digestive system working? Do you have frequent bouts of indigestion or an upset stomach? From my experience and many others, a tablespoon of organic apple cider vinegar in spring water is the best remedy to relieve both conditions. It ends indigestion by helping to digest your food and an upset stomach by eliminating what caused it. Plus, its prebiotics and probiotics help restore a healthy gut microbiota required for a healthy digestive system.

So the next time you get indigestion or an upset stomach, drink some as soon as possible; it usually works within minutes. It also helps relieve heartburn (see Tip 12 - Heartburn Remedy).

Food Poisoning Relief

Organic apple cider vinegar is also a great remedy to relieve food poisoning, a telltale sign that you consumed some bacteria or parasites. The next sign is usually diarrhea. Here its antibacterial and antiparasitic properties can quickly eliminate the root cause and help you feel better.

A friend, for instance, was once suffering from food poisoning and indigestion. He reluctantly drank a tablespoon in spring water and, to his astonishment, was cured in less than five minutes! I've seen this work many times as well.

Don't go on vacation without a bottle.

How to Buy

Most non-organic brands of apple cider vinegar are filtered (clear) and pasteurized, which significantly reduces their nutrients. Plus, they use non-organic apples that contain pesticides. Therefore, it is best to buy organic apple cider vinegar brands (e.g., Bragg, Fairchild) that instead use organic apples and are unfiltered (cloudy brown) and unpasteurized and have a brown sediment known as the "Mother" for it harbors a concentrated source of its nutrients. Shake well.

Dosage

Since organic apple cider vinegar contains acids, it's best to consume only one tablespoon at a time, around three times a day. That's all you need to help maintain vitality and a healthy immune response. Besides mixing it with spring water, add it to a glass of juice or a cocktail.

To help remain youthful and sick-free, don't go a day without a tablespoon.

Tip 4

Alcohol Health Benefits?

Perhaps what makes alcohol so appealing is its ability to boost dopamine and serotonin levels, two of your main feel-good neurotransmitters (a.k.a. chemical messengers). Studies have also found some potential health benefits of drinking alcohol in moderation or what is considered a few drinks a day. Many point to a positive link between moderate alcohol consumption and a lower risk of cardiovascular diseases and mortality than teetotalers because of alcohol's ability to reduce artery-clogging bad LDL (low-density lipoprotein) cholesterol and increase good HDL (high-density lipoprotein) cholesterol, which absorbs LDL cholesterol (and triglycerides) and sends it back to the liver to be flushed from the body.

For instance, a study published in the Journal of Clinical Lipidology found that overweight people who consumed a few drinks a day helped prevent dyslipidemia or elevated levels of LDL cholesterol and triglycerides (the most common form of fats) in the bloodstream. Over time, this condition significantly increases the risk of atherosclerosis.

Atherosclerosis, the narrowing and hardening of the arteries, is mainly caused by consuming foods high in unhealthy saturated fats and LDL cholesterol, which builds up plaque in the artery walls. And with this condition, plaque not only constricts normal blood flow, causing high blood pressure, it can also break off from an artery and cause a blood clot that could lead to a stroke or a heart attack. Although "alcohol consumption of up to 7 drinks/week at early middle age is associated with lower risk for future HF [heart failure], with a similar but less definite association in women than in men," according to the study, Alcohol Consumption and Risk of Heart Failure: the Atherosclerosis Risk in Communities Study, which included 14,629 participants. So alcohol may also help prevent a stroke or a heart attack by helping to prevent the buildup of artery plaque.

And if you are at a high risk for a blood clot or coronary problems, drinking alcohol with dinner may help lower your risk, according to the study, the Effect of Moderate Dose of Alcohol with Evening Meal on Fibrinolytic [Blood Clot] Factors. Researchers found "a decrease in risk of coronary [heart arteries] heart disease in moderate drinkers."

Brain Health Connection

Light to moderate drinking may reduce your age-related risk of dementia, according to the review, Moderate Alcohol Consumption and Cognitive Risk, which reviewed 143 scientific papers. Researchers found "Overall, light to moderate drinking does not appear to impair cognition in younger subjects and actually seems to reduce the risk of dementia and cognitive decline in older subjects." In addition, "Compared with abstention, consumption of 1 to 6 drinks weekly is associated with a lower risk of incident dementia among older adults," according to the study, Prospective Study of Alcohol Consumption and Risk of Dementia in Older Adults, which included 5888 participants 65 and older who drank beer, wine, or liquor.

This may be attributed to alcohol's potential ability to help your brain cleanse itself of toxins and waste products linked to dementia and Alzheimer's disease, according to the study, Beneficial Effects of Low Alcohol Exposure, But Adverse Effects of High Alcohol Intake on Glymphatic Function. Researchers "hypothesize that boosting of glymphatic [a waste pathway] function in combination with the reduction in GFAP [glial fibrillary acidic protein] expression might potentially contribute to the lowered risk for Alzheimer's disease and non-Alzheimer's dementia among individuals with habitually low but non-zero alcohol intake."

Longevity Connection

"Low levels of alcohol intake (1-2 drinks per day for women and 2-4 drinks per day for men) are inversely associated with total mortality in both men and women," according to the study, Alcohol Dosing and Total Mortality in Men and Women: An Updated Meta-Analysis of 34 Prospective Studies.

Furthermore, researchers "included 1,824 individuals between the ages of 55 and 65…[and found] compared to moderate drinkers, abstainers had a more than 2 times increased mortality risk, heavy drinkers had 70% increased risk, and light drinkers had 23% increased risk," according to the study, Late-Life Alcohol Consumption and 20-Year Mortality.

Heeding to Moderation

Although many other studies find that drinking alcohol (especially binge drinking) can cause significant health problems, such as cirrhosis of the liver and cancer by increasing free radicals; however, antioxidants help counteract them.

Nevertheless, as with many things in life, moderation is the key.

Disclaimer Time: If you don't drink, don't start for health reasons.

Tip 5

Healthier Cocktails

If you enjoy a few drinks a day, studies find it may contain some health benefits. Ironically, some mixers may potentially cause health problems if they contain refined sugar (see Tip 25 - Overcoming Sugar Addiction) or artificial sweeteners (see Tip 26 - Kicking the Artificial Sweeteners Non-Nutritive Habit).

For example, a large European cohort (group) study found that consuming just two or more sugar or artificially sweetened soft drinks a day increases your risk of mortality from all causes. Many soft drinks also contain phosphoric acid, which gives them their tangy flavor and protects against bacteria growth, but it also weakens your tooth enamel and is linked to causing kidney stones and disease.

In addition, refined sugar, artificial sweeteners, and high fructose corn syrup sweetened products are linked to non-alcoholic fatty liver disease (extra fat cells) that over time can also cause cirrhosis (scarring) of the liver.

What to do? A healthier solution to mixing a cocktail is to use "organic" mixers, juices, or teas. In contrast, they contain vitamins, minerals, and antioxidants that help counteract alcohol's free radicals and fight diseases. And according to USDA organic regulations, they cannot contain artificial sweeteners or high fructose corn syrup. Also look for brands without added sugars.

Organic Cocktail Examples

Whisky, Organic Green Tea & Raw Honey: Green tea and raw honey provide a healthy mix of antioxidants that help protect against free radicals and oxidative stress. Research finds that whisky also contains antioxidants.

Rum & Organic Grape Juice: Grapes contain potent antioxidants and anti-inflammatory properties that help protect against premature aging and chronic diseases. And rum (alcohol) reduces stress.

Screwdriver: Vodka & Organic Orange Juice: Orange juice is a great source of vitamin C, a powerful antioxidant that also contains antiseptic, antibacterial, and antiviral properties that help build your immune system. And a little alcohol also enhances your immune response.

Sea Breeze: Vodka, Organic Cranberry & Grapefruit Juice: Cranberries contain antioxidants and antibacterial properties that help prevent urinary tract infections by preventing the E. coli bacteria from attaching and multiplying on the urinary tract walls. Grapefruits also contain antioxidants and antibacterial properties.

Classic Bloody Mary: Vodka, Organic Tomato Juice & Celery: Tomatoes are a good source of potassium, an electrolyte that helps prevent and relieve a hangover. They're also a good source of the antioxidant lycopene, which helps prevent liver and brain cell damage. Celery also contains antioxidants and is a good source of natural sodium and other electrolytes that helps calm the nerves and relieve stress. A study found that vodka decreases oxidative stress in swine fed a "high-fat/cholesterol diet."

Your turn. March 24 is US National Cocktail Day, and May 13 is World Cocktail Day.

Tip 6

Red Wine's Potential Health Benefits

Red wine is known for its potential cardiovascular and longevity health benefits. Research finds that even "Among patients with established heart disease, moderate consumption of wine seems to be associated with lower incidence of CVE [cardiovascular events] and total mortality as compared with nondrinkers," according to the study, Wine Consumption and Risk of Cardiovascular Events After Myocardial Infarction [Heart Attack]: Results From the GISSI-Prevenzione Trial, which evaluated 11,248 Italian myocardial patients over seven years.

Moderate "consumption of red wine helps in preventing CVD [cardiovascular disease] through several mechanisms, including increasing the [good HDL] high-density lipoprotein cholesterol plasma levels, decreasing platelet aggregation, by antioxidant effects, and by restoration of endothelial [cell] function," according to the review, Red Wine: A Drink to Your Heart. The endothelial cells are flat (squamous) cells that resemble fish scales and line the interior surface of your blood vessels, known as the endothelium (membrane). Whereas a damaged endothelium is a benchmark for diagnosing oxidative stress, atherosclerosis, and cardiovascular disease.

Plus, the polyphenols found in red wine make blood

platelets less sticky, reducing your risk of a blood clot.

Potent Source of Polyphenols (Antioxidants)

Red wine's polyphenols include catechins, epicatechins, anthocyanins, proanthocyanidins, quercetin, and resveratrol. "Although the antioxidant property of red wines is correlated with their phenol content, no single compound sufficiently defines the total antioxidant capacity, because of the potential synergistic antioxidant effect of other compounds," according to the review, Molecular Properties of Red Wine Compounds and Cardiometabolic Benefits. In other words, they all work together. A glass of red wine contains approximately 200 mg of polyphenols, which depends on the type of grape and growing conditions. The RDA is around 1000 mg.

A bonus, the antioxidants found in red wine counteract the free radical effect of consuming alcohol, with a net antioxidant result, according to the study, Red Wine Consumption Increases Antioxidant Status and Decreases Oxidative Stress in the Circulation of Both Young and Old Humans. Researchers recruited "20 young (18–30 yrs) and 20 older ($\geq$ 50 yrs) volunteers…[and found] the consumption of 400 mL/day [13.5 ounces] of red wine for two weeks, significantly increases antioxidant status and decreases oxidative stress in the circulation."

The French Red Wine Paradox

The most famous wine study is Wine, Alcohol, Platelets, and the French Paradox for Coronary Heart Disease. Published in 1992, researchers found that the paradox or contradiction is that the French have a higher consumption of saturated fats than many other countries but still have a 40% lower risk of coronary heart disease likely due to their higher consumption of red wine's polyphenols. Many drink a glass or more a day.

Brain Health

Red wine's antioxidants also help protect your brain from oxidative stress, according to the study, Wine Polyphenols: Potential Agents in Neuroprotection. Researchers here found the "neuroprotective effects in in vitro [test tube] and in vivo [within the living] models of neurodegenerative disorders have been documented, and our own findings suggest that their mechanism of action involves their antioxidant activity, principally as scavenging intracellular ROS [reactive oxygen species] and inhibition of LDL oxidation."

Gut Health

Studies also find red wine's polyphenols increase the growth and diversity of beneficial gut bacteria while preventing the growth of pathogenic (disease-causing) bacteria.

Lung Health

"Red wine inhibits proliferation of lung cancer cells and blocks clonogenic [clone] survival at low concentrations," according to the study, Inhibition of Human Lung Cancer

Cell Proliferation and Survival by Wine. The researchers "data suggest that wine may have considerable anti-tumor and chemoprevention properties in lung cancer and deserves further systematic investigation."

Furthermore, "We show that endothelial damage, oxidative stress, vascular inflammation, and cellular aging were completely attenuated when red wine was consumed before smoking," according to the study, Red Wine Prevents the Acute Negative Vascular Effects of Smoking.

So smokers who drink should also drink red wine.

Oral Health

The polyphenols in red wine reduce the number of mouth bacteria that lead to tooth decay and gum disease, according to the study, Inhibition of Oral Pathogens Adhesion to Human Gingival Fibroblasts by Wine Polyphenols Alone and in Combination with an Oral Probiotic. These results "highlighted the anti-adhesive capacity of caffeic and p-coumaric acids as well as grape seed and red wine oenological extracts."

Red Wine vs. White Wine

Because white wine is mainly fermented from white grapes (and without the grape skins and seeds), it contains less antioxidants than red wine. Nevertheless, studies find that white wine is also heart healthy.

Red wine is also a good source of melatonin (found in grape skins), your body's natural sleep hormone. So a nighttime glass may help you sleep better while helping to keep your arteries clear of plaque.

Tip 7

Beer vs. Wine

Many studies suggest a few glasses of red wine is healthy. But what about beer's potential health benefits? How does it compare to wine?

For instance, "Beer, in contrast to wine and spirits, is a...source of B-vitamins and folate [needed to reduce high homocysteine levels], which might explain the result of lowest homocysteine plasma levels in the beer-preferring subgroup of our patients' sample and consequently the moderate degree of brain volume reduction," according to the study, Hippocampal [Two Hippocampus Memory Centers] Volume Loss in Patients With Alcoholism is Influenced by the Consumed Type of Alcoholic Beverage, which "included 52 patients with alcohol dependence." Elevated levels of the non-essential amino acid homocysteine is also linked to dementia. Although red wine's antioxidants also help protect against high homocysteine levels.

Beer also contains antioxidants. Hops (flowers from the Humulus lupulus plant), the most widely used ingredient in brewing beer, contains the polyphenol antioxidant xanthohumol, which has antioxidant properties similar to red wine's polyphenols in protecting against cardiovascular diseases and cancer. And malt (e.g., barley or wheat), the most widely used grain in brewing beer, also contains potent polyphenols. Plus, Brewer's yeast (e.g., Saccharomyces cerevisiae) that's required to brew beer is a good source.

According to the Phenol-Explorer: An Online Comprehensive Database on Polyphenol Content in Foods, the "Total polyphenol content in beer, as measured by the Folin method, varies between 12 and 52 mg/100 ml [3.4 oz], depending on the beer type. Ale beer and dark beer are richer in polyphenols (52 and 42 mg/100 ml respectively). Regular beer contains about 28 mg/100 ml total polyphenols. Alcohol free beer contains about 12 mg/100 ml polyphenols." And for wine the "Average total polyphenol content measured by the Folin method is 216 mg/100 ml for red wine and 32 mg/100 ml for white wine." In short, drinking a regular 12-ounce beer contains around 100 mg of polyphenols, which equals around a half glass of red wine.

The polyphenols found in wine and beer also help maintain a healthy gut microbiota by increasing beneficial gut bacteria and decreasing pathogenic bacteria.

And as with wine, beer helps lower bad LDL cholesterol and increases good HDL cholesterol, which is also a potent antioxidant, according to the review, Moderate Beer Intake and Cardiovascular Health in Overweight Individuals that included 21 men and 15 women with an average age of 48.3 ± 5.4 years. Researchers found that a "moderate intake of beer increases the anti-oxidative [antioxidant] properties of HDL and facilitates cholesterol efflux [outflow], which may prevent lipid [fat] deposition in the vessel wall."

Beer is also a good source of the mineral silica needed for the maintenance of your bones and to help produce collagen, the main structural protein.

Though "any healthy effects of wine and beer are greater

in combination with a healthy diet," according to the review, Wine, Beer, Alcohol and Polyphenols on Cardiovascular Disease and Cancer. For instance, "the health benefits associated with the Mediterranean diet, which combines moderate wine and beer consumption with a diet rich in fruits, vegetables and whole grains."

Tip 8

Health Concerns with Drinking Alcohol on an Empty Stomach

If you ever drank alcohol on an empty stomach, you have most likely felt that uneasy, sometimes painful sensation of alcohol rolling around in your stomach, which is nothing to brush off and keep drinking. The next time, use this as a telltale sign to consume some food before you drink more—and for good reasons. Drinking alcohol on an empty stomach can harm the cells of your stomach, kidneys, and liver, increasing your risk of organ damage such as cirrhosis of the liver: symptoms include jaundice, a yellowing of the skin and whites of the eyes.

But by lining or coating your stomach with a healthy meal before your first drink, you at least provide your organs with some protection. And since food helps to slow down alcohol's absorption rate in your bloodstream, you are less likely to experience the painful consequences of a prolonged hangover. In other words, the same amount of alcohol will still be metabolized, but with food in your belly, you'll hopefully be able to hold your booze better, prolong your organs' life, and beat most hangovers.

Hypertension Risk

Consuming alcohol without food also increases your risk of high blood pressure or hypertension, according to the study, Relationship of Alcohol Drinking Pattern to Risk of Hypertension. Researchers found "in a sample of 2609 white men and women from western New York, aged 35 to 80 years, and free from other cardiovascular diseases… [that] drinking outside meals appears to have a significant effect on hypertension risk independent of the amount of alcohol consumed."

So protect your body by eating something substantial before drinking alcohol.

Tip 9

Potential Problems with Drinking Beer (or Anything) Out of Aluminum Cans

Aluminum cans are interlined with a thin polymer lining to prevent aluminum toxicity from leaching into the beer (and potentially causing neurological disorders). Although they're not always 100% effective, especially if the can is damaged. Either way, your mouth still comes in contact with the metal.

An Aluminum-Alzheimer's Disease Link?

In 1901, Dr. Alois Alzheimer diagnosed a patient named Auguste Deter who was suffering from memory loss, delusions, aggression, and paranoia. After her death in 1906, he conducted an autopsy on her brain and found bundles of neurofibrillary (neuron fiber) "tangles" and clumps of amyloid (abnormal protein) "plaques" that are now known as the two hallmarks of Alzheimer's disease (AD), the most common type of dementia or the loss of cognitive functions.

But what causes the neurofibrillary tangles and amyloid plaques to form? Scientists believe AD is linked to genes, lifestyle, occupation, diet, and the environment. For instance, high levels of aluminum have been found in the brains of AD patients. Whereas "Al [aluminum] exposure promotes oxidative stress and amyloid deposition in the nervous tissue which results in neurodegeneration," according to the review, Aluminum Toxicosis: A Review of Toxic Actions and Effects.

And "Since 1911, experimental evidence has repeatedly demonstrated that chronic Al intoxication reproduces neuropathological hallmarks of AD," according to the review, Aluminum and Alzheimer's Disease: After a Century of Controversy, Is there a Plausible Link? This research recommends that "Immediate steps should be taken to lessen human exposure to Al, which may be the single most aggravating and avoidable factor related to AD."

Although "because the precise mechanism of AD pathogenesis remains unknown, this [Aluminum-Alzheimer's disease link] issue is [still] controversial. However, it is widely accepted that Al is a recognized neurotoxin, and that it could cause cognitive deficiency and dementia when it enters the brain and may have various adverse effects on CNS [central nervous system]," according to the review, Link between Aluminum and the Pathogenesis of Alzheimer's Disease: The Integration of the Aluminum and Amyloid Cascade Hypotheses.

Aluminum toxicity is also linked to myocarditis (inflammation of the heart muscle), multiple sclerosis, autism, breast cancer, fibrosis, bone diseases, pancreatitis, and diabetes. So it's wise to also avoid other aluminum-containing products such as aluminum cookware and utensils, aluminum foil, aluminum lined milk and juice cartons, packaged cheese slices, table salt, soy protein isolate, antacids, buffered aspirin, and antiperspirants and toothpaste not labeled aluminum-free.

It's also good to know what water source your favorite beer uses. According to the study, Aluminum and Silica in Drinking Water and the Risk of Alzheimer's Disease or Cognitive Decline: Findings From 15-Year Follow-up of the PAQUID Cohort, researchers analyzed the geographic exposure to aluminum and the mineral silica from 91 public water systems in southern France and found that "cognitive decline with time was greater in subjects with a higher daily aluminum intake from drinking water ($\geq$ 0.1 mg/day, $p = 0.005$) or a higher geographical exposure to aluminum. Using a Cox model [an analysis of survival data], a high daily intake of aluminum was significantly associated with an increased risk of dementia. Conversely, an increase of 10 mg/day in silica [commonly found in water] intake was associated with a reduced risk of dementia." How? Silica chelates (bonds) to aluminum and removes it from circulation. And since beer is a good source of silica (averages 15 mg in a 12-ounce beer), drink it out of a glass bottle, which ironically is mainly made from silica sand.

Plus, high-fiber foods and sulfur-containing foods such as cruciferous vegetables, onions, and garlic also help remove aluminum from your body. And vitamin E, the mineral selenium, and the spice turmeric especially helps protect against aluminum-induced free radicals and oxidative stress.

Another Can Concern: Bisphenol A (BPA)

The polymer lining of some aluminum beer cans are still made with the toxic chemical Bisphenol A (BPA), a popular building block of epoxy resins and polycarbonate plastic, which also leaches into products. It's been found in 93% of all Americans, according to the Centers for Disease Control and Prevention (CDC).

The BPA health concern is that it's also a well-known endocrine (hormone) disruptor linked to oxidative stress, miscarriages, early puberty, thyroid malfunctions, high blood pressure, obesity, diabetes, heart disease, brain damage, and cancer. Even very small amounts are harmful. So in 2012, the FDA banned the use of BPA in the manufacturing of baby bottles and sippy cups. But it's still used in some canned beers, canned foods, and polycarbonate plastic bottles (recycling code 7 indicates it contains BPA). It's also found in some imported products.

In addition, also avoid products that contain Bisphenol S (BPS), usually labeled BPA-Free. It's just as bad as BPA, if not worse. Besides similar health problems, researchers from the University of Guelph, Ontario, found BPS can depress or hinder a female mouse's heart function quicker than BPA. "In females BPS decreased left ventricular systolic pressure by 5 min, whereas BPA effects were delayed to 10 min." This is a significant health concern for women (and men) with cardiovascular problems such as high blood pressure.

To help counteract Bisphenol's toxicity, research recommends to consume antioxidant-rich fruits and vegetables and to drink green tea.

So it's not just what you drink, but also what you drink it out of. Anyway, doesn't beer taste better out of a glass bottle?

Tip 10

Hangover Prevention and Recovery Remedies

Hangovers are nothing new. Archaeologists have unearthed pottery with rice beer residues over 9,000 years old.

Why some people are more prone to hangovers than others usually depends on their genetic makeup. Historically, men seem to have a higher tolerance than women because of their larger body frame. But, of course, that's not always true: some women can drink men under the table and still be hangover-free.

Hangover Prevention Remedies

Here are some tips to help prevent a hangover:

- Eat first. You're less likely to get drunk on a full stomach since food slows down the rise of alcohol in the bloodstream. So, for example, eat a serving of fish or chicken with a sweet potato and salad. But avoid salty foods such as chips and pretzels for they make your body retain extra fluids.

- Take a 50 mg vitamin B complex before drinking and before bedtime. It helps prevent a hangover by metabolizing alcohol and reducing mental and oxidative stress. And since they are water-soluble vitamins, alcohol can create a deficiency that can heighten the effects of a hangover, such as headaches, dizziness, fatigue, memory problems, and the blues. Also Wernicke-Korsakoff Syndrome, a severe memory disorder, is caused by a thiamin (vitamin B1) deficiency as the result of chronic alcohol abuse or malnutrition. (See Tip 30 - Importance of Vitamin B Complex.)

- Take a 15 mg zinc supplement. It also helps prevent a hangover by metabolizing alcohol. And it protects against alcoholic liver disease. Although alcohol also lowers its levels. Good food sources include seafood, meat, nuts, and seeds.

- Drink a glass of spring water every hour. It helps dilute and flush out alcohol before it can settle in your head and cause a hangover. After all, your brain consists of approximately 75% water.

Hangover Recovery Remedies

The next time you have a hangover, here are some tips to help you feel better and recover quicker:

- Stay hydrated with spring water. It's required for regulating body temperature, transporting nutrients, and flushing out waste. Raw fruits and vegetables are also good sources of water.

- Consume protein-rich foods. They provide needed energy while helping to repair your body. Good sources include seafood, lean meat, poultry, eggs, and Brewer's yeast.

- Consume fiber-rich foods. They help restore and maintain healthy glucose (energy) levels. Good sources include fruits, vegetables, whole grain breads, beans, nuts, and seeds.

- Consume foods that contain the minerals potassium, sodium, calcium, and magnesium. They help relieve a hangover by restoring your electrolyte (electric charged) equilibrium. Good sources include bananas, oranges, avocados, tomatoes, celery, spinach, broccoli, beets, beans, and sweet potatoes.

- Take a 50 mg vitamin B complex. It improves mental and physical health.

- Take a 600 mg L-cysteine (or N-acetyl-L-cysteine) supplement, an amino acid found to help alleviate alcohol-induced headaches, nausea, anxiety, and stress. It also increases your glutathione levels needed to detoxify your liver and body. Good food sources include eggs, fish, poultry, beef, broccoli, onions, garlic, and Brewer's yeast.

- Do aerobic (cardio) exercises. According to researchers at the University of Colorado at Boulder, aerobic exercise may prevent and reverse the damaging effects of heavy drinking on your brain's white matter, which houses the nerve fibers (axons) that connect and transmit brain cell signals; its health is vital for a clear mind. Exercise also releases endorphins, one of your natural pain-relievers. Try aerobics, walking fast, jogging, or cycling for 20 minutes.

Tip 11

Milk "Liver Helper" Thistle

If you drink alcohol regularly, it's only natural to wonder from time to time: How's my liver holding out?

After your skin, your liver is your second largest organ. Weighing around three pounds and roughly the size of an NFL football, its many functions include detoxifying and purifying your blood, metabolizing and storing fats, proteins, vitamins, and minerals, and producing HDL cholesterol, digestive bile, and hormones (a.k.a. chemical messengers).

It's also perhaps the most resilient organ in your body. Research finds that you could cut off half of your liver and it can regenerate itself back to normal size within a month. So your liver is a workhorse that can take some abuse.

The Liver Friendly Plant (Herb)

The milk thistle plant is what nature made to help protect, cleanse, and rejuvenate your liver cells. You've most likely seen the milk thistle plant before. A member of the daisy family, it has green-prickly leaves with purplish-pink flower heads and grows in pastures and along roadsides.

According to the article, Milk Thistle: Early Seeds of Potential, the "Greek physician and botanist Dioscorides (40–90 AD) was the first to describe milk thistle's healing properties." Its "use can range from the mundane—e.g., fighting hangovers—to potentially life-saving for patients who have ingested poisonous mushrooms—particularly amanita [death cap] mushrooms, which release a specific toxic called amatoxin."

The key to its long medicinal success is a powerful flavonoid antioxidant called silymarin, which is found in its seeds. Silymarin protects your liver from free radicals and oxidative stress while enhancing liver regeneration. It also increases glutathione (master antioxidant) levels needed to detoxify your liver.

"Silymarin has [also] shown positive effects as supportive treatment in most forms of liver disease including cirrhosis and liver damage due to alcohol abuse. In clinical trials that included patients with cirrhosis, there was a significant reduction of liver-related deaths with silymarin treatment. The mechanism of action by which silymarin produces these clinical effects is attributed to its antioxidant activity," according to the review, Silymarin as Supportive Treatment in Liver Diseases: A Narrative Review.

Hence, milk thistle is considered the "gold standard" herb for treating liver disorders. In some countries, it's prescribed for hepatitis and cirrhosis of the liver. It also protects against non-alcoholic fatty liver disease, also known as the "teetaler's cirrhosis of the liver."

Dosage

If you feel you need some extra liver support, it's recommended to take around 200 mg of milk thistle extract once or twice a day. For the highest quality supplement, the label should state it's extracted or standardized to at least 75% silymarin.

And while helping to protect and regenerate your liver, milk thistle also boosts your immune system and mental clarity.

Tip 12

Heartburn Remedy

Heartburn, also known as acid reflux or backwash, got its name for the burning sensation it causes, although it has nothing to do with your heart muscle. It's a digestive issue caused by hydrochloric acid (a strong acidic acid needed to break down protein) irritating the lining of your esophagus or swallowing tube. And reoccurring bouts may be a sign of gastroesophageal reflux disease (GERD) or chronic heartburn, which increases your risk of esophagus cancer. So heartburn is not to be taken for granted.

Common Causes of Heartburn

A frequent cause of heartburn is a weak lower esophageal sphincter. Located in the lower part of your esophagus, the lower esophageal sphincter is a ring-like band of muscle fibers that connects to your stomach muscle and creates a high-pressure zone. Its primary job is to work as a one-way valve: opening to allow food to enter the stomach, then securely closing to prevent food and hydrochloric acid from exiting up into your esophagus. But being overweight or overeating can weaken the lower esophageal sphincter valve by adding extra pressure, causing it to open.

Or you may be consuming more acidic foods than alkaline foods. Acidic foods such as spicy, fatty, or fried foods can relax your lower esophageal sphincter, allowing hydrochloric acid to exit upwards.

Another cause is when your digestive system cannot digest food properly for the lack of digestive enzymes. Instead of breaking down food so it can enter the small intestine, where nutrients are absorbed into the bloodstream, the food is now stuck in your gut. Then its extra pressure opens the valve.

Even though your pancreas gland produces enough digestive enzymes to digest your food properly, these critical enzymes can be overwhelmed when your diet has a ratio of more cooked (dead) foods than raw (alive) foods such as fruits, vegetables, nuts, and seeds for their enzymes aid in healthy digestion. So anyone deficient in enzymes (internal or external) will eventually get heartburn.

Curing Heartburn

No matter what the cause, a quick remedy to cure and prevent heartburn is to drink a tablespoon of organic apple cider vinegar in spring water. Its digestive properties (e.g., enzymes, prebiotics, and probiotics) usually ends it within minutes.

Taking a digestive enzyme supplement also quickly ends heartburn by digesting your food. They are essential if you don't consume your daily share of enzyme-containing raw fruits and vegetables. Look for a standard enzyme supplement that contains the following key digestive enzymes:

- Protease for digesting protein
- Bromelain for digesting protein
- Amylase for digesting carbohydrates
- Lipase for digesting fats
- Cellulase for digesting fiber
- Sucrase for digesting sugar and starches

Carry around a few digestive enzymes pills for when you need them the most—like after eating a sausage and pepperoni pizza. (You'll be glad you did.)

These two remedies are also a much safer option than taking those expensive pharmaceutical heartburn pills (e.g., Purple Pill/Nexium) with their long list of harmful side effects. Total cost for relieving heartburn and improving your digestive health with a tablespoon of organic apple cider vinegar and an enzyme supplement: around 50 cents, and without any harmful side effects. According to friends and acquaintances who suffered for years from chronic acid reflux, these two remedies cured it, unlike the heartburn pills, which just temporarily eased their symptoms.

Although many will never get heartburn in the first place if they consume raw produce with every meal.

Tip 13

Naturally Getting "The Red Out"

When your eyeballs' tiny blood vessels become irritated and dilated, it increases blood flow that causes them to swell, making the sclera (white surface) of your eyes appear red.

How do you get the red out? With over-the-counter eye drops? In a pinch, they work well to relieve the appearance of red (bloodshot) eyes with vasoconstrictors that temporarily narrow the swollen blood vessels to constrict blood flow. But they also contain preservatives that are toxic to the surface of your eyes, such as benzalkonium chloride, a chemical that's known to cause dry eyes, reduce tear production, and damage cornea cells. Fortunately, there is a better temporary solution.

Preservative-free eye drops are available. To prevent spoilage (oxidation), look for drops packaged in single-use containers.

But either way, the increased blood flow that causes red eyes is usually a sign that your body is trying to repair a problem. And repeatedly constricting your eye's blood vessels with either type of eye drop may constrict your body's natural ability to correct this problem. So whichever one you use, save them for when you really need them, like driving home at night. And instead of using two drops per eye, use only one. You'll get the same results.

Another option is to turn to nutrition.

Red Eye Nutrition Remedies

Here are some nutrients that help get the red out while nourishing your eyes:

Vitamin A

Vitamin A is needed for clear eyes and good vision for it's the precursor to producing the chromoprotein rhodopsin, the "visual purple" pigment in your retinas that allows you to see in low light and at night. Therefore, a vitamin A deficiency causes night blindness. The best food sources include liver, cantaloupes, carrots, sweet potatoes, broccoli, kale, spinach, squash, and red bell peppers.

Vitamin B Complex

A deficiency of B vitamins also affects your eyesight, which can result in an increased sensitivity to light, blurred vision, and bloodshot eyes. Good sources include whole grains, beans, nuts, seeds, spinach, broccoli, lean meat, poultry, seafood, eggs, and Brewer's yeast. Or take a vitamin B complex supplement.

Mineral Zinc

After your inner ear, your eyes' retina contains the second highest concentration of zinc in your body. It protects against red eye oxidative stress and visual disorders including cataracts and macular degeneration. The best food sources include seafood, lean meat, eggs, beans, peas, nuts, and seeds. For extra eye insurance, take a 15 mg zinc supplement.

Eye Antioxidants Lutein and Zeaxanthin

The antioxidants lutein and zeaxanthin are mainly found in your eyes' retinas which senses light so you can see. And in your macula, the retinas' yellow spot that allows you to see in fine detail and in color. Its yellow color is even derived from their pigment.

Research finds they protect against oxidative stress and visual disorders including cataracts, macular degeneration, and retinal detachment. They also absorb blue light generated from computer screens, helping to prevent eyestrain and blurred vision.

Lutein and zeaxanthin are found in various carotenoid-containing produce such as carrots, squash, spinach, asparagus, kale, broccoli, bell peppers, parsley, peas, and corn. And egg yolks.

Other nutrients that help get the red out while nourishing your eyes include vitamin C, vitamin E, and omega-3 fatty acids, which are covered in more detail in the book.

Tip 14

Overcoming Baggy Dark Circles

Have too many late nights left you with more than red eyes? Do you also have baggy dark circles under your eyes? Has it reached a point they still won't go away even with a good night's sleep? Unlike when you were younger.

When baggy dark circles don't easily go away, you're probably lacking more than sleep. The skin located under your eyes is very thin, making it very sensitive to many disorders. And ironically, getting too much sleep may cause baggy dark circles.

The Usual Causes of Baggy Dark Circles

Besides a lack of sleep (or too much), consuming inflammatory foods or foods that rank high on the Glycemic Index (GI) is also linked to baggy dark circles. The GI is a numerical measurement of how quickly carbohydrates break down and raise your glucose or sugar levels. Whereas high-fiber foods rank low on the GI and low-fiber foods rank high. In other words, low-fiber foods such as white bread, white rice, and pastries break down quickly, which raises unhealthy glucose levels, increasing the inflammation linked to baggy dark circles. And high-fiber foods such as vegetables, whole grains, and beans break down slowly, which maintains healthy glucose levels, preventing the inflammation linked to baggy dark circles.

Consuming inflammatory foods is also linked to an imbalanced gut microbiome, causing skin microbiome disorders. Known as the "gut-skin axis," gut microbes (bacteria) imbalances are found to cause acne, atopic dermatitis, psoriasis, rosacea, and a puffy face and eyes. Hence, healthy skin also depends on a healthy gut.

Dark (blood) circles can also be caused by a lack of iron, folate (vitamin B9), or vitamin B12, which are required to make hemoglobin, a protein in your red blood cells that carries oxygen throughout your body. How are your iron and B vitamin levels? In a severe case, you could be borderline anemic (lacking red blood cells).

Another cause is dehydration; you may need to drink more healthy fluids. Or you may have fluid retention; how much table salt do you consume in a day? It causes your body to retain extra fluids, increasing overall blood pressure, including in the tiny capillaries (blood vessels) around your eyes, which can result in the swelling and puffiness of the skin below the eyes.

Allergies can also cause baggy (puffy) dark circles. Are you allergic to anything?

Poor circulation is also linked to baggy dark circles. How much weekly exercise do you get?

Diet Tips to Help Overcome Baggy Dark Circles

Here are some of the best diet tips to help prevent and overcome baggy dark circles:

- Stay hydrated by drinking a glass of spring water every few hours.

- Consume foods that contain calcium, which is also required to help build strong and healthy skin cells. Good sources include salmon, sardines, collard greens, turnip greens, kale, broccoli, sweet potatoes, oranges, beans, and almonds.

- Consume foods that contain iron, folate, and B12. Again, they are required to make hemoglobin and healthy red blood cells, which helps prevent dark circles. Good sources of iron include dark green lettuce, spinach, asparagus, peas, blackstrap molasses, lean beef, liver, poultry, and clams. (But avoid taking iron supplements unless menstruating because obtaining too much can cause oxidative stress.) Good sources of folate include romaine lettuce, spinach, asparagus, broccoli, black-eyed peas, whole grains, peanuts, beef liver, and seafood. Good sources of B12 include red meat, clams, oysters, salmon, trout, tuna, poultry, egg yolks, and kidney beans. Or take a B12 sublingual supplement; for best absorption, let it dissolve slowly under the tongue.

- Consume foods that contain vitamin A, which is required to help build and maintain firm skin. It also acts as a natural moisturizer that helps prevent dry, scaly skin. Good sources include carrots, sweet potatoes, apricots, cantaloupes, broccoli, Brussels sprouts, kale, and spinach.

- Consume foods that contain vitamin C. It's essential to make collagen (Greek for glue), which builds and holds your skin's molecular structure in place. Therefore, healthy skin contains high concentrations of vitamin C. Good sources include oranges, strawberries, lemons, limes, cantaloupes, kiwi, peppers, broccoli, Brussel sprouts, kale, spinach, tomatoes, and parsley.

- Consume foods that contain vitamin E. It protects cell membranes (lipids) from oxidative stress, reducing skin aging. It's also a natural skin moisturizer that reduces under eye bags. Good sources include wheat germ, almonds, hazelnuts, peanuts, sunflower seeds, avocados, olives, and olive oil. For extra skin insurance, take a 200 IU to 400 IU vitamin E mixed tocopherol supplement.

- Consume foods that contain omega-3 fatty acids, which are required to build healthy skin cell membranes. They also help prevent inflammation. Good sources include wild salmon, sardines, trout, cod, herring, clams, shrimp, avocados, broccoli, walnuts, and pumpkin seeds. (See Tip 49 - Omega Fatty Acids Build and Maintain a Healthy Brain.)

- Consume foods that contain the structural mineral silica. It improves your skin structure by increasing the production of collagen. Good sources include bananas, celery, cucumbers, green beans, bell peppers, asparagus, whole grains, and brown rice.

- Consume foods that contain vitamin K, required for healthy blood clotting, it also helps prevent and repair broken eye capillaries that can cause dark circles. Good sources include kale, spinach, collard greens, Brussels sprouts, broccoli, parsley, and romaine lettuce.

- Avoid inflammatory foods or foods high in fat, salt, sugar, or refined flour to maintain a healthy gut-skin microbiome. Instead, consume high-fiber (prebiotic) foods to nourish your beneficial gut bacteria (microbes). Good sources include vegetables, whole grains, beans, nuts, and seeds. Also consume fermented (probiotic) foods to increase your levels of beneficial gut bacteria. Good sources include sauerkraut, miso, pickles, yogurt, sourdough bread, and organic apple cider vinegar.

- Avoid table salt to prevent a retention of extra fluids, a leading cause of baggy eyes. Instead, consume foods high in natural sodium such as carrots, celery, spinach, parsley, beets, kelp, beans, and eggs. And when buying packaged foods, look for "no or low sodium (table salt) foods." (See Tip 24: Beating Table Salt's Deadly Addiction.)

- Avoid refined sugar (table sugar). It can deplete essential vitamins and minerals required to maintain healthy skin. Sugar can also bond with skin proteins and form advanced glycation end products (AGEs), a leading cause of wrinkles and sagging skin. Instead, get your natural sugar or glucose fix with fruits, vegetables, nuts, and seeds. (See Tip 25 - Overcoming Sugar Addiction.)

- Consume foods that contain the antioxidant alpha lipoic acid. Found in all your cells, it's known as the "universal antioxidant" because it is water-soluble and fat-soluble, meaning it protects the whole skin cell; inside and outside from inflammation and oxidative stress. It also helps prevent the formation of AGEs. Plus, it increases collagen production and protects it from breaking down. Good sources include Brewer's yeast, brown rice, organ meats, carrots, beets, broccoli, Brussels sprouts, spinach, tomatoes, and peas. For extra skin insurance, take a 600 mg alpha lipoic acid supplement.

- Take a 200 mg grape seed extract supplement. It's one of the best sources of proanthocyanidin antioxidants that strengthen your collagen and elastin connective tissues. (See Tip 19 - The Antioxidant Powers of Grape Seed "Youth" Extract.)

- Consume foods that contain the antioxidant superoxide dismutase. Often used in skin care products, it's well-known to protect skin from inflammation and free radicals, reducing your risk of wrinkles, bags, and age spots. Good sources include broccoli, Brussels sprouts, cabbage, peas, chickpeas, spinach, tomatoes, honeydew melon, cantaloupe, cashews, pumpkin seeds, wheat grass, barley grass, and Brewer's yeast.

- Consume less cooked and canned (dead) foods and more raw (alive) enzyme-containing foods such as fruits, vegetables, nuts, and seeds, which is a key to preventing skin aging.

- Exercise daily. It improves circulation, including in the tiny blood vessels around your eyes, helping to prevent baggy dark circles.

A healthy diet and exercise keeps the dermatologist away.

Tip 15

Naturally Relieving Coughs and Cottonmouth

Can't shake a cough? Or got cottonmouth? Here are some healthy ways to help quickly relieve both conditions.

Besides a cold or an underlining respiratory condition such as asthma, coughs are usually caused by mucus or other obstructions in your air passageways; cottonmouth or dry mouth by a lack of saliva, dehydration, or inhaling bad air. And if your tiny cilia hairs are damaged, this will allow more obstructions to enter your lungs, further irritating these conditions.

Your cilia hairs line your respiratory tract (airways and lungs). When working correctly, they catch mucus, bacteria, and foreign particles and discard them through your nose and mouth. But when damaged, you're more likely to have a dry throat, a hoarse cough, breathing problems, or other respiratory issues.

To help nourish your cilia hairs back to health and relieve other common causes of these problems, consume any 100% juice (e.g., grape, apple, black cherry, orange) or a lemon wedge and spring water. Their medicinal properties are found in their organic water, citric acid, vitamins, minerals, and antioxidants.

Another effective remedy is to drink a cup of green tea and raw honey. Their antioxidants and anti-inflammatory properties also help relieve these conditions.

For best results, first mix these drinks around in your mouth before slowly swallowing. And if you have throat pain or sores, gargling with a tablespoon of organic apple cider vinegar in spring water will deliver quick relief.

Also keep a glass of lemon and water covered on your nightstand for when you need relief in the middle of the night. (See Tip 36 - Lemon Aid.)

To help prevent future coughs and cottonmouth, try to determine what caused either in the first place. Then adjust your diet, lifestyle, or environment.

Tip 16

Apples Keep the Lung Doctor Away

Are you having breathing problems? Short of breath? Research finds that consuming five or more red apples a week can significantly improve your lung function, which is mainly attributed to the flavonoid antioxidant quercetin found in their skin or peel.

Quercetin also reduces a smoker's risk of lung cancer by 53%, according to the study, Dietary Quercetin, Quercetin-Gene Interaction, Metabolic Gene Expression in Lung Tissue and Lung Cancer Risk. Researchers found the "inverse associations for quercetin-rich foods were seen in both women and men, ever smokers, and were strongest in the heaviest smokers [a pack a day]."

For people with asthma, quercetin also acts as an anti-inflammatory that helps improve breathing. And for allergy sufferers, it contains antihistamine properties.

And like all flavonoids (plant defense compounds that contain antioxidants), quercetin helps regulate blood pressure by improving blood vessel functions. Other studies find that quercetin reduces the risk of colon, liver, pancreas, and breast cancer. Besides apples, quercetin is also found in berries, oranges, onions, broccoli, kale, asparagus, tomatoes, red wine, and tea.

Apples also contain other powerful antioxidants that

improve lung function, including anthocyanins, procyanidins, epicatechins, gallic acid, and vitamin C. They also contain a significant source of fiber that studies also find to improve lung function. A medium apple, for example, contains approximately 4.5 grams of soluble and insoluble fiber, or roughly 20% of the recommended daily allowance. Apples also contain protein, vitamin A, B vitamins, vitamin E, vitamin K, calcium, magnesium, potassium, copper, and iron.

Organic vs. Conventional Apples

It's best to buy organic apples because most non-organic or conventionally grown apples contain an average of four different pesticide residues, according to data from USDA Pesticide [Residue] Data Program.

Plus, organic apples contain a healthier balance of beneficial gut bacteria than conventional apples, according to the study, An Apple a Day: Which Bacteria Do We Eat With Organic and Conventional Apples? Researchers found that "Organic and conventional apples are occupied by a similar quantity of microbiota; consuming the whole apple includes an approximate uptake of 100 million bacterial gene copy numbers. However, freshly harvested, organically managed apples harbor a significantly more diverse, more even and distinct microbiota."

Red Apples vs. Green Apples

Because of their darker skin, red apples contain more antioxidants than green apples. Nevertheless, research finds green apples are also beneficial for your lungs and gut. So add both to your diet.

And since their antioxidants are mainly found in their skin, it's best to eat apples whole instead of peeling them. Plus, their flesh (insides) is also a source of antioxidants. Chewing apples whole also helps keep your teeth white for they also contain malic acid, a natural whitening (bleaching) agent often used in toothpaste. But avoid eating apple seeds for they contain small amounts of cyanide, a deadly poison that protects the seeds from predators.

The saying, "An apple a day keeps the doctor away," is still timely. The original quote is an 1866 Welsh proverb: "Eat an apple on going to bed and you'll keep the doctor from earning his bread."

For smokers, two organic apples a day may be their silver bullet.

Tip 17

Fruits and Vegetables for Smokers and Ex-Smokers

Research finds that your lungs have an amazing "self-cleaning ability" to heal and regenerate their cells and cilia hairs from smoking tobacco, especially with a healthy diet.

And "In current smokers, consumption of vegetables and fruits may reduce lung cancer risk, in particular the risk of [the deadly] squamous cell carcinomas," according to the study, Fruits and Vegetables Consumption and the Risk of Histological Subtypes of Lung Cancer in the European Prospective Investigation into Cancer and Nutrition, which included 478,535 participants from ten countries. Researchers found the "Risks of squamous cell carcinomas in current smokers were reduced for an increase of 100 g/day [approximately a cup] of fruit and vegetables combined."

The lung health benefits of consuming fruits and vegetables are mainly linked to their powerful antioxidants. For instance, according to the study, Inverse Association between Dietary Intake of Selected Carotenoids and Vitamin C and Risk of Lung Cancer, researchers found "several dietary antioxidants found in common food sources may protect against lung cancer, even among heavy smokers." In short, the antioxidant vitamin C found in oranges, lemons, and broccoli; the antioxidant lycopene found in tomatoes, watermelon, and pink grapefruits; the antioxidant beta-cryptoxanthin found in red bell peppers, mangos, and peaches; and the antioxidants beta-carotene and alpha-carotene found in apricots, carrots, and sweet potatoes—all showed significant protection against lung cancer in heavy smokers.

Although cigarette smoke depletes "a variety of carotenoid antioxidants, including beta-carotene," according to the study, Dietary Antioxidants and Cigarette Smoke-Induced Biomolecular Damage: A Complex Interaction. This is due to its "over 4700 chemical compounds including high concentrations of oxidants and free radicals present in both the gas phase and tar phase of cigarette smoke," according to the study, Oxidant/Antioxidant Imbalance in Smokers and Chronic Obstructive Pulmonary Disease [COPD].

Nevertheless, "fruit and vegetable consumption is inversely associated with chronic obstructive pulmonary disease and may explain why some smokers do not develop chronic obstructive pulmonary disease," according to the study, The Association Between Diet and Chronic Obstructive Pulmonary Disease in Subjects Selected From General Practice. Researchers found that a 10-year pack-a-day smoker who doesn't consume their daily share of antioxidant-rich fruits and vegetables significantly increases their risk of developing COPD, an umbrella term for emphysema and chronic bronchitis.

Fruits and Vegetables for Healthier Lungs

For healthier lungs, ideally consume produce with every meal. For instance, two fruits for breakfast, three vegetables for lunch, and five vegetables (salad) for dinner. And they're all lung healthy, especially apples, blueberries, black cherries, grapes, bananas, oranges, mangos, tomatoes, carrots, celery, broccoli, Brussel sprouts, kale, cabbage, cauliflower, asparagus, beets, sweet potatoes, mushrooms, corn, spinach, romaine lettuce, peppers, onions, and garlic. Plus, they're all good sources of fiber, which improves lung function.

Particularly for ex-smokers, consuming apples and tomatoes may help repair lung damage, according to the study, Dietary Antioxidants and 10-Year Lung Function Decline in Adults From the ECRHS Survey. Researchers found that their "antioxidants possibly contribute to restoration, following damage caused by exposure to smoking, among adults who have quit."

When possible, buy organic produce. They contain more nutrients and antioxidants because they're grown without chemical fertilizers and pesticides (see Tip 34: Organic Produce or Bust?).

Fruits and vegetables are lung medicine.

Tip 18

Vitamins for Smokers and Ex-Smokers

Studies find that the antioxidants vitamin A, vitamin C, vitamin E, and vitamin D improve lung function and help protect smokers and ex-smokers from lung disorders such as COPD and lung cancer.

Vitamin A

The antioxidant vitamin A, for instance, activates and increases your immune system's T cells (white blood cells) that guard against infections and chronic diseases. Therefore, "During moderate vitamin-A-deficiency, the incidence for diseases of the respiratory tract is considerably increased," according to the article, Importance of Vitamin-A for Lung Function and Development. It's "also responsible for the development of many tissues and cells as well as for the embryonic lung development."

Although smoking cigarettes depletes its levels, which is also linked to emphysema, according to the study, Vitamin A Depletion Induced by Cigarette Smoke Is Associated with the Development of Emphysema in Rats. Researchers found that benzo(a)pyrene, a common carcinogen in cigarette smoke, induces a vitamin A deficiency in rats, causing emphysema.

Nevertheless, vitamin A reduces the risk of COPD (emphysema and chronic bronchitis) by an estimated 52%, according to the study, Do Vegetables and Fruits Reduce the Risk of Chronic Obstructive Pulmonary Disease? A Case-Control Study in Japan, which included 278 COPD patients.

Vitamin A is a fat-soluble vitamin (your body stores it). So taking a high-dose supplement can be toxic rather than obtaining it from fruits and vegetables that contain high amounts because it must be first metabolized from its precursors (beta-carotene, alpha-carotene, or beta-cryptoxanthin), making it unlikely to cause toxicity.

Good food sources of vitamin A include carrots, sweet potatoes, apricots, cantaloupes, broccoli, Brussels sprouts, kale, spinach, liver, and herring. The RDA is 3000 IU, which equals approximately a carrot.

Vitamin C

Smoking also depletes vitamin C levels, a potent antioxidant that protects against lung disorders. Research has found "a protective role for vitamin C against the risk of obstructive airways disease and support the hypothesis that vitamin C may be an effect modifier for the adverse effects of smoking on the risk of obstructive airways disease," according to the study, Interaction of Vitamin C With the Relation Between Smoking and Obstructive Airways Disease in EPIC Norfolk. European Prospective Investigation into Cancer and Nutrition, a "population-based study of 3,714 males and 4,256 females aged 45-74 yrs."

And the "results from this meta-analysis suggest that a high intake of vitamin C might have a protective effect against lung cancer, especially in the United States. Dose-response analysis indicated that the estimated risk reduction in lung cancer is 7% for every 100 mg/day increase in intake of vitamin C [from fruits and vegetables]," according to the study, Association Between Vitamin C Intake and Lung Cancer: A Dose-Response Meta-Analysis.

Research also finds that vitamin C increases vitamin E levels in smokers, another vital line of defense against cigarette's toxins.

Vitamin C is a water-soluble vitamin that your body cannot produce. So smokers and nonsmokers need a plan to replenish it. Good food sources include oranges, grapefruits, lemons, strawberries, papaya, bell peppers, broccoli, Brussels sprouts, kale, and parsley. The RDA is 90 mg, which equals approximately a medium orange.

Vitamin D

Smoking tobacco also depletes the antioxidant vitamin D, the sunshine vitamin, which is also an essential nutrient to protect against lung disorders. For instance, a "Vitamin D deficiency was associated with lower lung function and more rapid lung function decline in smokers over 20 years in this longitudinal cohort of [626] elderly men. This suggests that vitamin D sufficiency may have a protective effect against the damaging effects of smoking on lung function," according to the study, Vitamin D Deficiency, Smoking, and Lung Function in the Normative Aging Study.

So "achieving an adequate vitamin D status should be a goal for everyone and may prove to be beneficial in the prevention of lung cancer," according to the review, Vitamin D: Potential in the Prevention and Treatment of Lung Cancer.

Furthermore, this "data indicate that vitamin D3 [the best source] may modulate the immune system and protect the lung from damage induced by cigarette smoke," according to the study, Effect of Vitamin D3 on Lung Damage Induced by Cigarette Smoke in Mice.

Vitamin D is also a fat-soluble vitamin. To reach healthy levels, the options are to get some weekly sunshine, take a vitamin D3 supplement, or consume vitamin D-rich foods. The current RDA is 800 IU, which equals approximately 3.5 ounces of wild salmon. Other food sources include sardines, herring, oysters, and eggs.

Vitamin E

The antioxidant vitamin E is one of the first lines of defense against cigarette smoke by protecting cell membranes (lipids) from lipid peroxidation (oxidative stress). And a "Higher vitamin E status, as measured by serum alpha-tocopherol concentration, as well as repletion of a low vitamin E state, was related to decreased lung cancer risk during a 28-year period," according to the study, A Prospective Study of Serum Vitamin E and 28-Year Risk of Lung Cancer, which included 22,781 male smokers.

In addition, the "results from this meta-analysis suggest that a high intake of vitamin E might have a protective effect against lung cancer," according to the study, Dietary

Vitamin E Intake Could Reduce the Risk of Lung Cancer: Evidence From a Meta-Analysis, which reviewed eleven studies involving 4,434 lung cancer cases.

And as with other vitamins, "cigarette smoke depletes plasma of vitamin E...[therefore] cigarette smoking does increase vitamin E requirements in humans," according to the study, Cigarette Smoke Alters Human Vitamin E Requirements.

Good food sources of vitamin E include wheat germ, almonds, hazelnuts, peanuts, sunflower seeds, avocados, olives, and olive oil. The RDA is 22 IU, which equals approximately a handful of mixed raw nuts and seeds.

For extra lung insurance, research suggest smokers (or anyone exposed to air pollution) should also take a vitamin E supplement. Vitamin E is a complex fat-soluble vitamin that contains eight fatty molecules: four tocopherols and four tocotrienols, commonly labeled "mixed tocopherols." This supplement delivers vitamin E's full antioxidant health benefits versus taking the more widely sold dl-alpha tocopherol supplement. Smokers should consider taking 200 IU to 400 IU a day, a dosage range recommended for disease prevention and treatment.

Tip 19

The Antioxidant Powers of Grape Seed "Youth" Extract

Hundreds of studies have been devoted to researching the health benefits of grape seeds, which are rich in polyphenol antioxidants, including one of the best sources of proanthocyanidins.

"Scientific studies have shown that the antioxidant power of proanthocyanidins is 20 times greater than vitamin E and 50 times greater than vitamin C," according to the review, Polyphenolics in Grape Seeds-Biochemistry and Functionality Extensive. Researchers also found "its antioxidant effect to bond with collagen, promoting youthful skin, cell health, elasticity, and flexibility."

Proanthocyanidins are able to cross-link (bond) to stabilize and strengthen collagen and elastin, the two main anti-aging proteins. Collagen, the most abundant protein in your body, is a strong structural protein that gives your skin its strength and firmness. Whereas elastin (elastic) is a stretchy protein that allows your skin to stretch and bounce back to its original shape. Together, they maintain the overall structural integrity of the connective tissues that support your skin, joints, blood vessels, organs, and muscles. Thus, grape seed extract helps build and maintain healthy connective tissues.

Proanthocyanidins also help prevent the mineral degradation of your dentin (yellow) collagen, preventing your teeth from turning yellow caused by losing its protective enamel or covering. They also strengthen composite fillings.

Blood Pressure and Artery Health

Grape seed extract's proanthocyanidins also help maintain healthy blood pressure levels. "It is widely recognized that oxidative stress is implicated in the pathogenesis of hypertension…[and] overwhelming evidence from in vitro experiments suggests that grape seed extract has an antioxidant property that can protect cells from ROS [reactive oxygen species]-mediated DNA damage," according to the meta-analysis, The Impact of Grape Seed Extract Treatment on Blood Pressure Changes.

Research also finds that its proanthocyanidins help prevent arteriosclerosis or the hardening of your arteries. For example, 146 patients diagnosed with carotid artery (neck blood vessel) plaques took 200 mg of grape seed extract per day and significantly reduced their plaque size that otherwise could have progressed into atherosclerosis, according to the study, Beneficial Clinical Effects of Grape Seed Proanthocyanidin Extract [GSPE] on the Progression of Carotid Atherosclerotic Plaques. The researchers' results found the "plaque score (10.9% decrease after six months, 24.1% decrease after 12 months and 33.1% decrease after 24 months)." They also found that eventually "the carotid plaque can disappear after treatment with GSPE." Plaques are mainly formed by a buildup of saturated fats, LDL cholesterol, and calcium deposits.

Memory Health

Its proanthocyanidins also help improve and protect your memory. Studies find it's beneficial for your brain's hippocampus (where memories are formed) by increasing neurogenesis (the birth of new brain cells) and by protecting them against oxidative stress (free radicals).

In another study, researchers caused ischemia (restricted blood flow) in rats to impair their memory. Then, afterward, treated them with grape seed extract, which significantly helped to regain and improve their memory. They concluded that the free radical scavenging powers of its polyphenols exhibit long-term potential for helping to maintain short- and long-term memories.

Grape seed extract may also help prevent and treat Alzheimer's disease, according to researchers at Mount Sinai School of Medicine in New York. They found that after five months of treatment, mice given 200 mg a day of grape seed extract had 30% to 50% less clumping of the amyloid plaques that cause Alzheimer's disease.

Cancer Prevention

Grape seed extract (GSE) is also a potential insurance policy against cancer. "Pre-clinical studies have established strong GSE efficacy against prostate, colon, lung, breast, skin, and other cancers," according to the study, Differential Effects of Grape Seed Extract Against Human Colorectal Cancer Cell Lines: The Intricate Role of Death Receptors and Mitochondria. "Importantly, GSE mediated cell death efficacy was found to be specific against CRC [colorectal cancer] cells as it exhibited no toxicity in normal colon epithelial cells," which are the cells that line the internal and external surfaces of your organs.

Other research finds that grape seed extract kills cancer cells without harming healthy cells, which is the biggest downside of chemotherapy and radiation; plus, it also helps to prevent their deadly free radicals from causing oxidative stress, according to the study, The Role of Grape Seed Extract in the Treatment of Chemo/Radiotherapy Induced Toxicity: A Systematic Review of Preclinical Studies.

And grape seed extract not only kills cancer cells but also helps prevent them from growing, according to the study, the Generation of Reactive Oxygen Species by Grape Seed Extract Causes Irreparable DNA Damage Leading to G 2 /M Arrest and Apoptosis Selectively in Head and Neck Squamous Cell Carcinoma Cells [HNSCC]. These "findings show that GSE targets both DNA damage and repair and provide mechanistic insights for its efficacy selectively against HNSCC both in cell culture and mouse xenograft [tissue or organ transplant]."

On top of that, grape seeds' proanthocyanidins "exhibited selective cytotoxicity [cell death] toward selected human cancer cells, while enhancing the growth and viability of normal cells," according to the study, Free Radical Scavenging, Antioxidant and Cancer Chemoprevention by Grape Seed Proanthocyanidin [GSP]: An Overview. Therefore, these "results demonstrate that GSP may serve as a novel therapeutic intervention against carcinogenesis [cancer formation]."

Lung Health

For people with asthma, research shows there's "no more gasping for air with grape seed extract." Its proanthocyanidins clear airways by reducing inflammation and free radicals.

For smokers, grape seeds' proanthocyanidins can reduce their risk of lung disorders such as COPD and lung cancer. It can also end smoker's cough.

Even More Health Benefits

Grape seed extract also helps prevent obesity by improving fat metabolism. It also increases beneficial gut bacteria while decreasing unhealthy bacteria induced by a long-term high-fat diet. And it improves liver function in patients with non-alcoholic fatty liver disease. Plus, it protects the kidneys from oxidative stress and premature apoptosis (programmed cell death to eliminate unwanted and damaged cells).

Other studies find that grape seed extract helps maintain strong bones, prevents and relieves arthritis (inflammation), reduces leg swelling due to prolonged sitting, and helps wounds heal faster.

In addition, grape seed extract prevents bacterial infections including Campylobacter and the superbug MRSA (Methicillin-resistant Staphylococcus aureus). And it stops fungal infections such as Candida.

It may be the most versatile external antioxidant ever.

Purchasing and Dosage

Grape seed extract supplements should be standardized to

at least 90% polyphenols or (oligomeric) proanthocyanidins. Research suggests taking 100 mg to 400 mg per day. I started taking 100 mg daily in 1997 and since have noticed firmer skin, healthier lungs, and a clearer mind.

Taking grape seed extract is considered safe. After all, it's just made from grape seeds. Although it can thin your blood (reducing your risk of a blood clot), but if taking blood thinners, first check with your doctor.

Grape seed extract also protects against skin cancer. Try not to sunbathe without the "youth" supplement.

Tip 20

Hot Peppers Healthy Buzz

When it comes to the health benefits of consuming hot peppers—the hotter, the better—ideally to the point you sweat a little. That's how you know they're really working, making them also a hangover remedy by helping to sweat out the after-effects.

Hot peppers' heat buzz comes from its active compound called capsaicin, which is also a powerful antioxidant found in all hot peppers such as cayenne, chili, tabasco, and habanero. It's renowned for creating a natural flow of heat energy that improves blood flow (circulation) while increasing energy levels. Capsaicin can't take the place of exercise for increasing blood flow, but in a pinch, it might be the next best thing.

This is also a key to how your trillions of cells receive their daily nourishment. You can eat right, but if you lack healthy blood flow, it can hinder the ability to circulate nutrients properly throughout your body.

Hot peppers' capsaicin also helps maintain healthy blood pressure levels by improving the function of your endothelium (the endothelial cells that line the interior surface of your blood vessels), according to the study, Activation of TRPV1 by Dietary Capsaicin Improves Endothelium-Dependent Vasorelaxation and Prevents Hypertension. Researchers "hypothesized that dietary capsaicin chronically activates TRPV1 [the capsaicin receptor that regulates body temperature], which contributes to the vascular [blood vessel] benefits."

Increases Longevity

Hot peppers also extend your life span, according to the study, Consumption of Spicy Foods and Total and Cause-Specific Mortality: Population Based Cohort Study, which included 199,293 men and 288,082 women aged 30 to 79 years. Researchers found "significant inverse associations between spicy food consumption and total and certain cause-specific mortality [cancer, ischemic heart diseases, and respiratory diseases]."

And "Adults who consumed hot red chili peppers had a 13% lower hazard of death, compared to those who did not," according to the study, The Association of Hot Red Chili Pepper Consumption and Mortality: A Large Population-Based Cohort, which included 16,179 participants, 18 years or older.

Liver Health and Weight Control

According to the European Association for the Study of the Liver, hot peppers help prevent liver damage by reducing the activation of cells that cause liver fibrosis or scar tissue.

Hot peppers also help manage your weight by enhancing energy levels and metabolism.

Stomach Ulcers and Hot Peppers Debate

After decades of scientific debate, it's now recognized that peptic ulcers (open sores on your stomach lining) are not caused by consuming hot peppers. Instead, they are caused by the Helicobacter pylori bacteria. And ironically, hot peppers' capsaicin contains antibacterial properties that inhibit the growth of this bacteria (and others). But if you have an ulcer, it's best to avoid hot peppers until cured to prevent any further inflammation.

Dosage

Consume one chili pepper or a tablespoon of cayenne pepper a day. That's all it takes. Add some to your food or put some in your beer.

Capsaicin also comes in a supplement. But you'll miss out on its full heat benefits if it has to first dissolve in your stomach. Remember that the digestive process begins in your mouth. Once capsaicin touches your tongue and saliva, it immediately enters the bloodstream, giving you that instance rush of heat energy throughout.

Consuming hot peppers also stimulates the release of endorphins, your body's natural painkillers that resemble opiates such as morphine in their ability to relieve pain and produce a sense of well-being. Surprisingly, your body releases endorphins after consuming hot peppers because it thinks your mouth is on fire and needs relief!

Tip 21

Sweet Potatoes: A Perfect Munchie Food

Too often, people have a hard time finding a healthy and tasty snack. Even with all the natural fast food options, too many still end up buying one that contains cavity-causing table sugar, blood pressure-raising table salt, or artery-damaging saturated fats. So read food labels carefully; your longevity may depend on it.

One healthier option is a sweet potato, a health-conscious cure for the munchies. It satisfies both your hunger and sweet tooth with a potent dose of nutrients that lift and sustain your energy levels—just the opposite of what many fast food snacks do to your body.

Sweet potatoes are also a quick snack to make if you slice one into small pieces and steam for around seven minutes.

Health Benefits

Sweet Potato's health benefits include "antioxidative, hepatoprotective, anti-inflammatory, antitumor, antidiabetic, antimicrobial, antiobesity, antiaging effects," according to the study, Chemical Constituents and Health Effects of Sweet Potato.

This is attributed to their outstanding source of plant protein, dietary fiber (soluble and insoluble), natural sugars, complex carbohydrates, calcium, potassium, B vitamin choline, vitamin C, and the antioxidants anthocyanin, phenolic acid, and beta-carotene, the main precursor to making the antioxidant vitamin A.

Sweet potatoes are one of the best sources of beta-carotene; therefore, they contain high levels of vitamin A. One medium orange sweet potato, for instance, contains over four times the recommended daily allowance. Though, once again, when your body receives natural sources of vitamin A instead of from a supplement source, it's unlikely to cause toxicity.

Here's how to tell if you are low on vitamin A: walk into a dark room and turn on a light. If it takes a long time to focus, there's a good chance your deficient. You can also tell when you are driving at night and someone turns on their bright lights and it becomes hard to focus. Excessive eye blinking is another telltale sign, as is dry skin. If concerned, request a vitamin A test from your doctor.

Ironically Sweet Potatoes Are Low in Sugar

Contrary to their name, sweet potatoes are low in sugar. A medium one only contains about seven grams. And since they are also high in fiber (four grams in a medium one), it makes them a complex carbohydrate food, which helps maintain healthy glucose levels.

Whereas white potatoes are also low in sugar (two grams in a medium one) but low in fiber (two grams) and high in white potato starch (thirty grams) versus an orange sweet potato (eight grams). As with refined white sugar and processed carbs, white potato starch is a simple carbohydrate that quickly breaks down, causing unhealthy glucose (sugar) spikes. According to the Glycemic Index, white potatoes rank higher than refined white sugar!

A Long Tradition of Longevity

Okinawa, Japan has one of the largest populations in the world of centenarians (100-year-olds or older). A link to their longevity is their long tradition of consuming sweet potatoes. They prefer purple sweet potatoes, which have a similar nutritional profile to orange sweet potatoes. The main difference is that purple sweet potatoes are higher in starch and anthocyanin (pigment) antioxidants and orange sweet potatoes are lower in starch and higher in beta-carotene (pigment) antioxidants. Ideally, add all types of sweet potatoes to your diet.

What Happens After Eating a Sweet Potato

After you consume a sweet potato, several healthy events occur inside your body. First, while satisfying your sweet tooth, it increases healthy glucose levels, your primary energy source. Then its B vitamin choline helps you think clearer and feel better for it's the precursor to producing acetylcholine, a key neurotransmitter for improving focus, learning, memory, and a sense of well-being. While this is happening, its antioxidants are protecting your body from free radicals and oxidative stress. And its antioxidant vitamin A is also protecting your eyesight while building your immune system. Plus, its soluble fiber is providing vital food for your beneficial gut bacteria (microbes) while its insoluble fiber is helping to sweep your colon clean. High-fiber foods also give you that full feeling, curing the munchies.

How to Purchase, Store and Cook

Look for sweet potatoes that are firm and without mold. To increase their shelf life, store in a cool, dry, dark place. Though it's not advised to refrigerate them for they will spoil faster.

To steam, cut into small pieces and steam for about seven minutes. But don't peel them because their skin is rich in protein, fiber, vitamins, minerals, and antioxidants.

To bake, preheat oven to 350 degrees and cook for 45 to 60 minutes, depending on how soft you like them. For an even healthier snack, add some lemon juice and olive oil. And spice them up with some cayenne pepper.

Sweet potatoes are a healthy snack or meal.

Tip 22

Garlic and Your Health

Garlic may not be one of the best foods to consume before going out on the town (for obvious reasons), but it's one of the best foods to consume to help recover from a long night—it's a healthy rush of detoxifying energy.

Garlic has been revered for over 5,000 years. In Egyptian culture, for instance, it was fed to the pyramid workers to increase their strength and endurance. It was also given to the original Greek Olympic athletes, making it perhaps the first "natural performance-enhancing supplement." Hippocrates is also known to prescribe it to fight fatigue, lung disorders, and parasites.

Since those times, thousands of studies have been devoted to researching this little bulb and its medicinal powers that are mainly credited to its sulfur properties, especially allicin, which gives garlic its pungent smell and taste.

Allicin is garlic's natural defense against pests. For you, it guards against viruses, fungi, bacteria, and parasites. It's also a powerful antioxidant and chelator that detoxifies heavy metals (e.g., aluminum, cadmium, cobalt, mercury, and lead), preventing potential organ damage. It also boosts your powerful internal antioxidants glutathione, superoxide dismutase, and catalase to protect against oxidative stress.

Cancer Protection Plus

Consuming garlic protects against stomach, colorectal, esophageal, prostate, ovarian, breast, and lung cancer. For instance, a "protective association between consumption of raw garlic and lung cancer has been observed in this present study with a clear dose-response pattern, suggesting that raw garlic consumption may potentially serve as a chemopreventive [cancer prevention] agent for lung cancer," according to the study, Raw Garlic Consumption as a Protective Factor for Lung Cancer, A Population-Based Case-Control Study in a Chinese Population, which included 1,424 lung cancer cases.

"Several mechanisms have been presented to explain cancer chemopreventive effects of garlic-derived products. These include modulation in activity of several metabolizing enzymes that activate and detoxify carcinogens and inhibit DNA adduct formation, antioxidative and free radicals scavenging properties and regulation of cell proliferation, apoptosis and immune responses," according to the study, Cancer Chemoprevention with Garlic and its Constituents.

Garlic also helps to maintain healthy blood pressure levels. Research finds that your red blood cells convert garlic's sulfur properties into hydrogen sulfide gas, which causes blood vessels to relax and widen.

It also reduces your risk of cardiovascular diseases by lowering levels of bad LDL cholesterol. Plus, it protects your liver cells from alcoholic liver disease and nonalcoholic fatty liver disease caused by a high-fat diet. And it guards against colds.

Other Nutrients

Garlic also contains B vitamins, vitamin C, manganese, calcium, potassium, phosphorus, selenium, iron, copper, and tryptophan, the amino acid that enables the production of the mood-enhancing neurotransmitter serotonin.

Best to Consume Garlic Raw

When you cook garlic, it destroys most of its allicin and other nutrients; so it's best to consume it raw. And higher amounts of allicin are produced after a garlic clove is chopped or crushed and exposed to oxygen for around 10 minutes.

One way to have it both ways is to cook with some garlic, then after your meal is done, add some raw garlic. Ideally, try to consume one to two garlic cloves a day. To help relieve garlic breath, chew on some fresh parsley or spearmint.

Medical Warning: Garlic naturally thins your blood, which protects against blood clots, but if you are taking blood thinners, scheduled for surgery, or pregnant, first check with your doctor.

Tip 23

What's the Deal with Red and Processed Meat?

Red meat is a great hangover remedy for it provides that much-needed full feeling while helping you rebound with its good source of protein, B vitamins, and zinc.

Although there are many downsides to consuming too much red meat or processed meat, which is considered more than three servings a week. Research has repeatedly found that it increases your risk of obesity, diabetes, non-alcoholic fatty liver disease, cardiovascular diseases, premature mortality, and cancer.

A serving size is around three ounces or what can fit into the palm of your hand. But consuming just two and a half ounces (76 grams) "a day" of red or processed meat increases your risk of colorectal cancer by 20%, according to the study, Diet and Colorectal Cancer in UK Biobank: A Prospective Study, which included half a million men and women from the United Kingdom.

Women should also know that lowering processed meat consumption is needed to prevent breast cancer, according to the study, Red and Processed Meat Consumption and Breast Cancer: UK Biobank Cohort Study and Meta-Analysis. Researchers found that "Over a median of 7 years follow-up, 4819 of the 262,195 women developed breast cancer. The risk was increased in the highest tertile (>9 g/day) [e.g., a slice of bacon] of processed meat consumption."

And men should also know that lowering red and processed meat consumption is needed to maintain a healthy sex life, according to the study, Meat and Meat-related Compounds and Risk of Prostate Cancer in a Large Prospective Cohort Study in the United States, which included 175,343 men aged 50-71 years. Researchers found that "Red and processed meat may be positively associated with prostate cancer via mechanisms involving heme iron, nitrite/nitrate, grilling/barbecuing, and benzo[a]pyrene [a PAHs carcinogen formed by high-temperatures]."

Red Meat's Ingredient Concerns

One of the main health concerns with consuming too much red meat is its artery-clogging saturated fats and bad LDL cholesterol that increase your risk for atherosclerosis, the hardening of the arteries. A 12-ounce sirloin steak, for example, contains approximately 19 grams of saturated fats and 312 mg of total cholesterol—not good news considering the maximum recommended daily allowance for saturated fats is 20 grams and 300 mg for cholesterol. As a result, "Greater red and processed meat consumption was associated with an unhealthy pattern of biventricular [heart chamber] remodelling, worse cardiac function, and poorer [stiffer] arterial compliance," according to researchers from the Queen Mary University of London who studied the MRI scans of 19,408 UK Biobank participants. They also found "In contrast, greater oily fish consumption was associated with a healthier cardiovascular phenotype and better arterial compliance."

Red meat's heme iron is another health concern. Even

though heme iron absorbs much better than the non-heme iron mainly found in plant foods, consuming "too much" generates reactive oxygen species (ROS free radicals) that cause oxidative stress, increasing your risk of premature aging and cancer. (On the other hand, a plant's source of non-heme iron also contains polyphenol antioxidants that protect against oxidative stress.)

Another health concern is that consuming red meat creates a byproduct called trimethylamine N-oxide (TMAO) that forms when your gut bacteria break down its nutrients carnitine, choline, and lecithin. TMAO promotes blood clotting, increasing your risk of a stroke and a heart attack. It also promotes oxidative stress, increasing your risk of atherosclerosis by aging the endothelial cells that line the interior surface of your blood vessels. The good news is that a compound called 3,3-dimethyl-1-butanol found in olive oil, balsamic vinegar, and red wine inhibits TMAO's formation. Garlic and plant polyphenols also inhibit TMAO.

Processed Meat's Ingredient Concerns

In 2015, after evaluating over 800 cancer studies, the World Health Organization (WHO)'s International Agency for Research on Cancer (IARC) classified red meat as a probable carcinogen and processed meat as a carcinogen! They found that a 50 gram (1.7 ounce) daily serving of processed meat increases your risk of colorectal cancer by 18%.

In addition, a 2019 Harvard University study found that "Increasing total processed meat intake by half a daily serving or more was associated with a 13 percent higher risk of mortality from all causes." Processed meats include hot dogs, sausages, bacon, corn beef, beef jerky, salami, pepperoni, and some deli meats.

The main health concern with consuming most processed meats, besides their saturated fats, cholesterol, and heme iron, is that they contain sodium (salt) nitrate or sodium nitrite, which are used as curing agents (preservatives) and color and flavor enhancers. Though after digested, they can form carcinogens called nitrosamines that damage your cells' DNA, increasing the risk of colon, stomach, rectal, pancreatic, prostate, and breast cancer.

Consuming sodium nitrite also generates reactive nitrogen species (RNS free radicals) that increase your risk of lung cancer and COPD, helping to explain why some non-smokers develop these conditions.

Whereas sodium nitrate is also linked to bipolar disorder by altering healthy gut bacteria, according to the study, Nitrated Meat Products are Associated with Mania in Humans and Altered Behavior and Brain Gene Expression in Rats. Researchers "found that a history of eating nitrated dry cured meat but not other meat or fish products was strongly and independently associated with current mania."

Some brands, however, now offer processed meats without sodium nitrate or sodium nitrite, which is currently allowed by the USDA to be labeled: No Nitrates or Nitrites Added, or Uncured. These brands mainly use non-organic celery powder (surprisingly allowed by USDA Organic regulations) as a natural curing agent or preservative replacement, although it naturally contains nitrates (as with some other vegetables). And non-organic celery powder is higher in nitrates because conventional celery is usually grown with synthetic nitrogen fertilizer. So when buying processed meats, look for brands that use "organic celery powder," which is lower in nitrates. Also look for brands that add vitamin C (ascorbic acid); research finds it inhibits the formation of nitrosamines. And when consuming processed meats, also consume vitamin C-rich foods such as oranges, strawberries, lemons, cantaloupes, peppers, broccoli, spinach, and tomatoes. Or take a 100 mg vitamin C supplement.

Healthier Alternative: USDA Organic Certified Meat

Factory-farmed cattle (roughly 70% of US cows) are routinely exposed to pesticides, heavy metals, and other environmental pollutants, which tend to collect in their tissues and in yours after you digest them.

They are also given antibiotics to control the growth of harmful bacteria. But this practice is also linked to antibiotic resistance or the birth of superbugs, increasing the risk of transmitting drug-resistant bugs to humans. And to increase cattle size, factory farmers inject synthetic growth hormones such as testosterone and estrogen, which are linked to increasing the risk of colon, prostate, breast, and lung cancer.

The healthier alternative is to purchase USDA organic certified meat, which bans the use of synthetic antibiotics and growth hormones and requires livestock to be fed an organic diet and have access to organic pastures.

Organic meats cost more, but worth it to prevent polluting your body with the cocktail of toxins and drugs found in factory-farmed cattle. Research also finds that organic (grass-fed) cattle tastes better and contains around

50% more omega-3 fatty acids than factory-farmed (grain-fed) cattle.

The Healthiest Way to Cook Red Meat

The healthiest way to cook red meat is at medium (or less) temperature. The health concern with cooking at higher temperatures is that it creates (more) harmful compounds called advanced glycation end products (AGEs) that increase your risk of premature aging and chronic diseases. AGEs are formed by a process called the Maillard Reaction (named after French chemist Louis Camille Maillard) that begins with glycation, the bonding of sugar molecules to proteins or lipids. They are "responsible for the 'browning' of tissue seen with aging as well as the 'browning' of food during cooking," according to the book Ryan's Retina (Sixth Edition) Chapter, Diabetic Retinopathy: Genetics and Etiologic Mechanisms.

Cooking at high temperatures also creates carcinogens called heterocyclic amines (HCAs) that form when meat is overcooked (e.g., when meat is charred) and polycyclic aromatic hydrocarbons (PAHs) carcinogens that form when meat absorbs hot smoke from a grill or a hot pan.

But you can help inhibit the formation of AGEs, HCAs, and PAHs by marinating or seasoning red meat with the antioxidants found in extra virgin olive oil, vinegar, garlic, lemons (vitamin C), tea, turmeric (curcumin), cayenne pepper, oregano, sage, rosemary, thyme, basil, or black pepper. After all, red meat is a hangover savior.

Tip 24

Beating Table Salt's Deadly Addiction

It's hard to beat table salt's addiction for it activates your opioid receptors, increasing feelings of pleasure. No surprise it's abundantly found in top-selling foods such as chips, hot dogs, sausages, bacon, deli meats, pizzas, tacos, burritos, soups, and most fast food meals. Just try eating them without it.

The US Food and Drug Administration's recommended daily allowance (RDA) for table salt is 2300 mg a day or one teaspoon. And 1500 mg a day if you have high blood pressure. Nevertheless, the US Centers for Disease Control and Prevention finds that most Americans consume over 3400 mg a day, which leads to many avoidable health problems.

Table Salt's Health Problems

Table salt is a refined salt (approximately 40% sodium and 60% chloride) that's linked to an increased risk of strokes, cardiovascular diseases, atrial fibrillation (irregular heartbeat), a weakened immune system, an imbalanced gut microbiota, memory loss, migraines, depression, hearing loss, diabetes, obesity, gallstones, kidney stones, kidney disease, cataracts, prostate disease, erectile dysfunction, brittle bones, and arthritis. In addition, a "higher frequency of adding salt to foods is associated with a higher hazard of all-cause premature mortality and lower life expectancy," according to the 2022 study, Adding Salt to Foods and Hazard of Premature Mortality, which included 501,379 UK participants. So table salt should be required to contain a "health warning label."

Table salt is most recognized, however, for causing high blood pressure or hypertension, also known as the silent killer because most victims have no symptoms. Too much table salt in your diet causes this condition by disrupting your kidneys' job of regulating a healthy balance of minerals and water for it attracts and holds water, increasing the volume of blood flowing through your blood vessels, which in turn raises your blood pressure levels. Over time, this extra pressure damages the blood vessel walls (endothelium), making them more likely to develop plaque deposits and stiffen.

And it doesn't take much. Research finds consuming just a few tablespoons of table salt a day significantly raises your blood pressure. This extra pressure also damages your heart muscle by enlarging it, according to the study, Association of Estimated Sodium Intake With Adverse Cardiac Structure and Function. Researchers found that high blood pressure is responsible for over 60% of deaths from strokes and over 50% from heart disease. And as with heart problems, consuming too much salt also leads to chronic kidney problems by overworking them and damaging their tiny blood vessels and nephrons (filters), allowing fluid and waste products to build up in the body.

Although table salt can also cause oxidative stress that damages the blood vessel walls leading to "arterial stiffness independent of blood pressure," according to the review, Vascular Effects of Dietary Salt. Researchers found that your internal antioxidant "Superoxide dismutase (SOD) is important for scavenging superoxide [free radicals] and a high salt diet has been shown to reduce SOD expression and activity," leading to oxidative stress and cardiovascular problems.

Salt's induced oxidative stress may also impair your memory. Researchers found "that a HS [high salt] diet in mice could impair both short and long-term memory, probably due to disturbed synaptic plasticity in the hippocampus," according to the article, a High Salt Diet Impairs Memory-Related Synaptic Plasticity via Increased Oxidative Stress and Suppressed Synaptic Protein Expression.

Salt is also linked to dementia. Researchers here found that the "Avoidance of excessive salt intake and maintenance of vascular health may help to stave off the vascular and neurodegenerative pathologies that underlie dementia in the elderly," according to the article, Dietary Salt Promotes Cognitive Impairment Through Tau Phosphorylation.

Getting Your Natural (Real) Sodium

Relying on table salt as your primary source of sodium may create a natural sodium deficiency. There is sodium in table salt, but not the natural kind your cells require to flourish, refined or not. What about unrefined sea salt? Sea salt is an organic unrefined salt that contains sodium and other minerals. It's, however, not any healthier because it still contains 98% sodium chloride (table salt is 99.9%); therefore, they both cause the same bodily harm. This also applies to Himalayan salt, which is also 98% sodium chloride.

On the contrary, the natural sodium your body requires is found, for instance, in lettuce, celery, and carrots. This is the true sodium electrolyte, also known as the "youth mineral," because it helps to keep your joints limber and flexible—just the opposite of what sodium chloride does to them.

Your body also requires natural sources of sodium for healthy fluid balance, blood pressure, heart functions, nerve impulses and transmissions, muscle functions, and metabolism. And for maintaining healthy kidneys, liver, and brain.

RDA for Natural Sodium

The FDA's RDA for sodium is calculated on table salt and measured by a teaspoon. But they should also measure it by foods high in natural sodium. For example, a medium mixed vegetable salad (e.g., lettuce, spinach, celery, carrots, broccoli, beets, and a hardboiled egg) equals approximately 500 mg of natural sodium, which is the estimated real RDA of sodium for adults.

Though, unlike table salt (sodium chloride), there's basically no limit to consuming natural sources of sodium. The best sources include celery, carrots, lettuce, spinach, beets, broccoli, parsley, kelp, and beans.

And because of its high alkalinity, consuming natural sodium lowers acidity levels, helping you to recover quicker from a hangover.

Repairing and Protecting Your Body From Table Salt

First, toss out your salt shaker. Then to help repair its damage to your blood vessels and organs, research recommends consuming foods that contain vitamin C, potassium, calcium, and magnesium, such as oranges, bananas, broccoli, and green leafy vegetables.

And when you consume foods high in salt also consume foods that contain superoxide dismutase, the important antioxidant that salt reduces. Good sources include broccoli, Brussels sprouts, cabbage, peas, chickpeas, spinach, tomatoes, honeydew melon, cantaloupe, cashews, pumpkin seeds, wheat grass, barley grass, and Brewer's yeast.

Also consume 100% grape juice. Its anti-inflammatory properties and antioxidants help protect your body from salt binges. For example, a study from the University of Michigan Health System found that rats fed a high salt diet with grape powder had "lowered blood pressure and improved cardiac function; reduced systemic inflammation; reduced cardiac hypertrophy, fibrosis, and oxidative damage; and increased cardiac glutathione."

To help beat your table salt cravings, switch to healthy spices like cayenne pepper, turmeric, curry, parsley, and oregano, which contain vitamins, minerals, and antioxidants that also help repair your body. Over time, hopefully, you'll crave these spices over table salt, as studies suggest.

Tip 25

Overcoming Sugar Addiction

Refined white sugar, also known as sucrose or table sugar, satisfies the sweet tooth and provides a quick burst of energy. But it also comes with many reasons why to find a better way to get your sweet fix, especially to help save your skin and teeth.

Overcoming its addiction, of course, is not easy. Those refined white sugar crystals are as addictive as hard drugs for they ignite your reward pathways, causing a chemical dependency. Sugar also disrupts your leptin hormone (chemical messenger) that lets you know when you're full and to stop eating.

Nutrition Problem

Sugar's health concerns start with stripping (refining) sugarcanes of their vitamins, minerals, amino acids, and fiber to create the end product: 99.5% pure sucrose. And it's not only deficient in nutrients, research finds sugar can also deplete nutrients from your body.

The refining process, however, produces an outstanding byproduct called blackstrap molasses. It's low in sucrose (most has been refined out) and high in calcium, potassium, and iron. But, unfortunately, it's not as popular as refined sugar.

Sugar's Main Health Concerns

Studies find that regularly consuming refined sugar increases your risk of oxidative stress, premature aging, cardiovascular diseases, tooth decay, obesity, kidney diseases, liver diseases, inflammatory bowel disease (colitis), diabetes, depression, and dementia. It also decreases the growth of beneficial gut bacteria, harming the health of your gut microbiota needed for a healthy digestive system.

Refined sugar also harms your mitochondria, the powerhouses of your cells, resulting in less energy. But since refined sugar ranks high on the Glycemic Index, it's one of the best ways to instantly spike your blood sugar levels to energy highs. But this type of sugar high wears off quickly. Thus, the sugar rush becomes the sugar crash, leading to the sugar blues.

It's estimated that many Americans consume over 60 pounds of refined sugar a year. It's no wonder why some are falling apart—mentally and physically—they're being crippled by sugar addiction.

Sugar's Premature Aging Connection

Sugar causes premature aging by taking a toll on your connective tissues, the collagen and elastin proteins that maintain its firmness and elasticity. And unchecked, sugar can cause deep wrinkles and a sagging jawline known as "sugar sag."

This condition is linked to sugar causing oxidative stress

(a free radical and antioxidant imbalance) and glycation, the process where sugar molecules bond to proteins or lipids and form harmful brownish compounds called advanced glycation end products (AGEs). AGEs are well-known to bond (cross-link) with your collagen and elastin proteins (tissues) and permanently alter their structure by turning them stiff and brittle, eventually leading to wrinkles and saggy skin. In other words, protein linkages are replaced by glucose, impairing normal tissue functions. And a high sugar diet accelerates glycation, causing more AGEs to form in your skin. A study published in the British Journal of Dermatology found that the AGEs' skin damage "generally arises after 35 years, then increases rapidly with intrinsic [natural] ageing." In addition, an increased accumulation of AGEs in human tissues is also linked to diabetes, kidney diseases, liver damage, eye diseases, atherosclerosis, cardiovascular diseases, COPD, breast cancer, and Alzheimer's disease. If concerned, an AGEs test is available.

Fortunately, you have natural ways of inhibiting the formation of AGEs with your internal antioxidants glutathione and alpha lipoic acid, which also helps to lower blood sugar levels. To boost them, consume foods that increase their levels such as broccoli, Brussels sprouts, kale, spinach, sweet potatoes, tomatoes, and Brewer's yeast. And with your sugar binges, take a 600 mg alpha lipoic acid supplement, which also increases your glutathione levels. But it's not recommended to take glutathione supplements. A randomized, double-blind, placebo-controlled clinical trial (the "gold standard" of epidemiological studies) by the Bastyr University Research Institute, Kenmore, WA, found that glutathione supplements do "not improve glutathione status, nor reduce markers of oxidative stress in healthy adults."

In addition, the antioxidant vitamins A, C, and E and the antioxidants found in fruits and vegetables also help inhibit the formation of AGEs.

The Number One Cause of Tooth Decay

Refined sugar fuels an acidic environment in your mouth, allowing cavity-causing bacteria (mostly Streptococcus mutans) to flourish by devouring the sugar surrounding your enamel. This is the number one cause of cavities and tooth decay. And the degree of tooth damage depends on how long sugar remains in contact with this bacteria. So to help prevent cavities and tooth decay, it's important to brush your teeth soon after consuming anything that contains refined sugar, such as cokes, cakes, cookies, chocolate, or ice cream.

And drink green tea. It contains a natural source of fluoride and the polyphenol antioxidant epigallocatechin-3-gallate (EGCG) that research finds to inhibit the growth and formation of the Streptococcus mutans bacteria.

Overcoming Sugar Addiction

To help overcome sugar addiction, avoid buying refined white sugar in bulk and products that contain it. Also avoid its many disguises such as brown sugar, invert sugar, turbinado sugar, organic sugar, and raw sugar. Then, over time, these sugars will taste too sweet because your taste buds have learned (again) to like the healthier natural sugars found in fruits, vegetables, whole grains, and nuts. These foods also stabilize your blood sugar levels for their sugars are wrapped in fiber, creating a healthy slow rise in blood sugar levels that provides sustained energy instead of just a quick sugar fix.

Once you cut back on table sugar, expect healthier blood sugar levels, clearer thinking, less aging, and more energy.

Tip 26

Kicking the Artificial Sweeteners Non-Nutritive Habit

The cheap alternative to table sugar is artificial sweeteners, a.k.a. non-nutritive sweeteners, which are also highly addictive (comparable to hard drugs) and hard to avoid since many packaged foods and beverages contain them (or high fructose corn syrup). As a result, many have unwittingly experienced some of their side effects, including cottonmouth, digestive problems, headaches, anxiety, weight gain, mental confusion, and depression.

Their Telltale Labels

The popularity of artificial sweeteners is driven by the public's desire for products low in sugar and calories to help them control their weight. So foods or beverages labeled diet, low-calorie, sugar-free, or zero-sugar most likely contain at least one as their primary sweetener.

This tricks people into believing that they can consume all they want without gaining weight. But just look around; this mindset is obviously not working—the USA and other parts of the world are more obese than ever. Research finds they are a prime culprit.

Food companies also add them to their products because

they're all inexpensive, very sweet (need to add less), and blend well with other product ingredients. The six FDA approved artificial sweeteners are Saccharin (Sweet'N Low), Sucralose (Splenda), Aspartame (NutraSweet, Equal), Acesulfame Potassium (Sweet One, Ace-K), Neotame, and Advantame. Who knows what they will come up with next? After all, they are a multi-billion dollar business—but at the expense of our health.

A Brief History

For the most part, the discovery of artificial sweeteners was by accident.

Saccharin, the first artificial non-nutritive sweetener, was discovered in 1879 by chemist Constantin Fahlberg. While researching a new coal derivative, he accidentally got some on a slice of bread he was eating and found it was 300 to 500 times sweeter than table sugar.

Likewise, Aspartame (180 to 200 times sweeter than table sugar) was discovered in 1965 by chemist Jim Schlatter. While working on an ulcer treatment, he accidentally got the compound on his fingers and then licked one to pick up a piece of paper. Thus, another artificial sweetener was born! This is also how Acesulfame potassium (200 times sweeter than table sugar) was discovered in 1967 by chemists Harald Jensen and Karl Clauss. While researching a chemical compound Clauss licked his finger.

And in 1976, Sucralose (600 times sweeter than table sugar) was discovered by chemists Leslie Hough and Shashikant Phadnis. Phadnis confused the words "testing" and "tasting" and tasted a compound 600 times sweeter than sugar.

Furthermore, Neotame (7,000-13,000 times sweeter than table sugar) was discovered in 1992 by chemists Claude Nofre and Jean Marie Tinti. And Advantame (20,000 times sweeter than table sugar) was discovered in 2008 by Ajinomoto, a food and biotech company.

Another popular sweetener is High Fructose Corn Syrup (1.5 times sweeter than table sugar) that instead is considered a processed sweetener. Although its health risks are similar to artificial sweeteners. It was discovered in 1957 by chemists Richard Marshall and Earl Kooi. It's now mainly made from GMO Roundup Ready corn.

Their Main Health Concerns

Artificial sweeteners are linked to increasing your risk of cardiovascular diseases, strokes, cancer, and dementia. And drinking just two or more artificially (or table sugar) sweetened beverages a day is "positively associated with all-cause deaths in this large European cohort; the results are supportive of public health campaigns aimed at limiting the consumption of soft drinks," according to the study, Association Between Soft Drink Consumption and Mortality in 10 European Countries, which included 451,743 participants.

They're also linked to obesity and metabolic syndrome (MetS). Researchers found that "individuals who consumed at least one soft drink per day had a higher prevalence of MetS, than non-consumers," according to the study, Diet Soft Drink Consumption is Associated with the Metabolic Syndrome: A Two Sample Comparison. Metabolic syndrome, a combination of obesity, high blood sugar, high blood pressure, high triglycerides, and high LDL cholesterol levels, significantly increase your risk of diabetes and cardiovascular diseases.

Consuming products that contain high fructose corn syrup is also linked to obesity and metabolic syndrome, especially since your body makes fat from fructose more readily than from other forms of sugar. For instance, Princeton University researchers fed high fructose corn syrup to male rats and found they gained 48% more weight and body fat (triglycerides) than rats fed table sugar (sucrose). And as with human metabolic syndrome, they also had more stomach fat. High fructose corn syrup also causes weight gain by slowing down your metabolism.

Artificial sweeteners and high fructose corn syrup can also accumulate in your liver tissues and cause non-alcohol fatty liver disease or extra fat cells. They also increase your risk of kidney disease. And they can also cause gut microbiota disorders by decreasing the number of beneficial gut bacteria.

How to Avoid

Artificial sweeteners and high fructose corn syrup are routinely added to soft drinks, energy drinks, flavored waters, bottled teas, breads, cereals, salad dressings, yogurts, protein bars, candy bars, and many other products. So read labels carefully before buying.

An alternative is to buy USDA certified organic foods, which are not allowed to contain artificial sweeteners or high fructose corn syrup.

Tip 27

Hold the Canola Oil

Consuming foods that contain canola oil is yet another health concern that's hard to avoid. It's routinely added to breads, crackers, potato chips, protein bars, salad dressings, mayonnaises, margarines, and many other products. And some restaurants are also using it to cook their food.

Canola oil is made from the seeds of the rapeseed plant, which are naturally high in erucic acid (around 50%), a monounsaturated fatty acid that's linked to health problems such as myocardial lipidosis, the fatty degeneration of the heart muscle. Nevertheless, rapeseeds are bred to contain the FDA's requirement of 2% or less of erucic acid; otherwise known as food-grade low erucic acid rapeseed (LEAR) oil.

And since 1997, most conventional canola oil is made from the seeds of the GMO canola plant (a.k.a. canola seeds), a genetically modified version of the rapeseed plant bred to resist Roundup's deadly herbicide glyphosate. Though besides erucic acid's health problems, research finds that ingesting GMOs (glyphosate) kills beneficial gut bacteria and may cause cancer. Surveys find that more than 70% of Americans want GMO foods banned, also known as "Frankenfoods."

Canola Oil Processing Concerns

Processing canola oil begins with crushing the GMO rapeseeds or canola seeds and then soaking them in the neurotoxin hexane, a derivative of petroleum used to extract the oil. Then (as with most industrial oils) it goes through a chemical refining, bleaching, degumming, and deodorization process where it's steamed (distilled) at high temperatures (200 degrees plus) to remove hexane and other odors that affect the smell and taste. However, according to the paper, the Characterization of Canola Oil Extracted by Different Methods Using Fluorescence Spectroscopy, chemical "Refining methods largely remove vitamin E, carotenoids and chlorophylls during bleaching and deodorization processes. Refining process renders canola oil a hydrogenated mess of trans fatty acids and their consumption may lead to heart problems, blood platelet abnormalities, increased cancer risk and free radical damage."

So much for the health claim that canola oil is low in unhealthy fats and a good source of healthy omega-3 fatty acids, which can't withstand processing at high temperatures. Rather canola oil is high in omega-6 fatty acids that creates an omega-3 fatty acid imbalance problem linked to causing inflammation, arthritis, heart disease, obesity, cancer, and neurological disorders. For instance, according to the study, Effect of Canola Oil Consumption on Memory, Synapse and Neuropathology in the Triple Transgenic Mouse Model of Alzheimer's Disease. Researchers "found that chronic exposure to the canola-rich diet resulted in a significant increase in body weight and impairments in their working memory."

Instead, canola oil must be cold-pressed to claim it's a good source of omega-3 fatty acids, but it still contains some erucic acid. You can find cold-pressed (GMO and organic) canola oil at some stores, but it's not highly practiced because it's more expensive. So most of the canola oil found on grocery store shelves and used by the food industry is made by the standard chemical manufacturing process, which besides erucic acid and glyphosate, also retains some hexane.

And as it may also apply to humans, research found that stroke-prone rats fed canola oil significantly decreased their antioxidants superoxide dismutase, catalase, and glutathione levels, which caused oxidative stress and shortened their life span. Research also finds it creates a vitamin E deficiency in piglets.

How to Avoid

Many food companies use canola oil because it's a cheap alternative to the more expensive oils like olive oil. So if a food label lists canola oil along with other oils that may be used in the manufacturing or ingredients of this product (a standard labeling term), it most likely contains canola oil.

Other chemically manufactured oils (vegetable oils) to avoid include corn oil, cottonseed oil, sunflower oil, safflower oil, and soybean oil.

Hold the canola oil and reach for cold-pressed extra virgin olive oil, which many studies find is joint, heart, and brain healthy.

Tip 28

Soy Health Alert

In 1996, the Monsanto company (now Bayer) introduced Roundup Ready (glyphosate resistant) GMO soybeans. Today, over 90% of the US soybean crop plants GMO soybean seeds. The soy food industry claims that soy helps lower cholesterol levels, reduces the risk of heart disease, builds strong bones, and fights cancer. Soy milk and tofu, for instance, are two of their top sellers. Other foods, from protein bars to baby formulas, contain another soybean form called soy protein isolate.

Although in 2017 the FDA proposed to revoke the 1999 soybean health claim: "A total of 25 grams of soy protein a day, as part of a diet low in saturated fat and cholesterol, may reduce the risk of heart disease." They found that "For the first time, we have considered it necessary to propose a rule to revoke a health claim because numerous studies published since the claim was authorized in 1999 have presented inconsistent findings on the relationship between soy protein and heart disease." And we're still waiting for them to act.

Soybean's Anti-Nutrient Problem

Soybean milk, tofu, edamame, and some other packaged soy foods use "unfermented soybeans" that contain anti-nutrients the bean uses as a defense mechanism to repel or inhibit predators. But when ingested, these anti-nutrients disrupt your digestive system's functions by inhibiting your ability to absorb nutrients properly.

Their anti-nutrients include protease and trypsin enzyme inhibitors that inhibit your protease and trypsin digestive enzymes from properly breaking down protein, reducing protein absorption. And phytate (phytic acid) that contains chelating (bonding) properties that inhibit minerals such as calcium, magnesium, iron, copper, and zinc from properly absorbing. Therefore, consuming unfermented soybeans can create nutritional deficiencies.

You can, however, reduce soybeans' anti-nutrients by sprouting or fermenting them. For instance, the soy foods miso, tempeh, and tamari usually use "fermented soybeans." But, either way, they're still not a complete source of protein.

Soybean's Protein Problem

Soybeans are not a complete source of protein because they're deficient in the essential sulfur-containing amino acid methionine (although it is added to some products). Lacking a complete source of protein is linked to premature aging, fatigue, depression, weak bones and muscles, brittle nails, and thin hair. In other words, you age more when you lack a complete source of protein.

Soybean's Reproduction Problem

Other research finds that soy increases the risk of reproductive problems. A Harvard University study, for instance, found that consuming half a serving of soy food a day (e.g., a cup of soy milk) lowers sperm count and may play a role in male infertility (most likely by inhibiting zinc's absorption required for healthy reproduction).

Soybeans also contain phytoestrogens (plant hormones) known as isoflavones that can interfere with a women's hormonal balance by mimicking estrogen, the female hormone necessary for sexual and reproductive health. But too much is linked to infertility and cancers of the uterus and breast.

Soybean's Thyroid Problem

Unfermented soybeans are a king of goitrogen or thyroid gland-disrupting foods for their isoflavones (e.g., genistein) inhibit your absorption of iodine, the key mineral required to synthesize its vital hormones. Your thyroid gland, the butterfly shaped endocrine gland located in the lower part of your neck, releases hormones that regulate bodily functions such as breathing, heart rate, body temperature, energy metabolism, and body weight.

Though if you have an iodine (hormone) deficiency, your body has a natural way of letting you know by forming a goiter, an enlargement of the gland.

Soy Protein Isolate Health Problems

Soy protein isolate is now the main source of protein found in many protein powders, protein bars, baby formulas, and veggie burgers.

Its health concerns begin in the manufacturing process. To make most soy protein isolate, soybeans are soaked in hexane (to separate its oil from protein) and acid-washed in aluminum tanks. Hence, hexane (a neurotoxin) and aluminum (linked to Alzheimer's disease) is found in the final product. Plus, it's spray-dried at high temperatures, which forms cancer-linked nitrites while reducing its amino acids.

It also contains mineral-inhibiting phytates and genistein.

Soybean Oil Health Problems

Also avoid soybean oil (chemically manufactured vegetable oil) that is unfortunately added to almost all brands of mayonnaises and salad dressings. It's high in omega-6 fatty acids that increase your risk of heart disease, obesity, diabetes, and fatty liver disease. And most soybean oil is partially hydrogenated, a process that forms artery-clogging trans fats.

Researchers from the University of California, Riverside also found that soybean oil may also cause genetic changes in your brain linked to neurological disorders, such as anxiety, depression, autism, and Alzheimer's disease.

Tip 29

Celery Health

As a hangover remedy, celery ranks high on the list with the help of the Bloody Mary cocktail. Its supply of organic water and other nutrients helps you rebound quicker. Even Hippocrates prescribed it over 2,000 years ago to help cleanse the kidneys and calm the nerves.

Overall, research finds that consuming celery promotes vitality while reducing stress, inflammation, high blood pressure, and your risk of joint, kidney, liver, lung, and heart problems.

Celery's Nutrients

Celery's nutrients include organic water, fiber, vitamin A, B vitamins, vitamin C, vitamin K, sodium, potassium, calcium, magnesium, manganese, phosphorus, copper, zinc, silica, and antioxidants. For instance, "Celery, because of compounds such as caffeic acid, p-coumaric acid, ferulic acid, apigenin, luteolin, tannin, saponin, and kaempferol, has powerful antioxidant characteristics, to remove free radicals," according to the study, A Review of the Antioxidant Activity of Celery. Researchers also found that "Celery can prevent cardiovascular diseases, jaundice, liver and lien diseases, urinary tract obstruction, gout, and rheumatic disorders." Its antioxidant apigenin has also been found to stop the growth of cancerous tumors.

Mental Health

Celery contains around 95% water that's essential for mental health by increasing blood flow to your brain and keeping it hydrated. And for an extra mental boost, celery contains the amino acid tryptophan, the precursor to producing the neurotransmitter serotonin that increases your sense of happiness and well-being.

Maintains Strong Bones and Skin

Have you noticed how a celery stalk resembles the shape of a human bone? Coincidence or not, research finds that its mineral silica increases your bone density and strength. It also improves the structure and firmness of your skin.

How to Purchase

Look for firm celery stalks and purchase organic celery for non-organic or conventional celery contains a variety of health-damaging pesticides.

And as with most vegetables, it's best to consume celery raw to obtain its maximum health benefits. A few stalks a day is ideal.

Tip 30

Importance of Vitamin B Complex

Vitamin B complex is known as the digestive vitamin, the energy vitamin, the anti-stress vitamin, the brain vitamin, and the youth vitamin.

Research finds you can age more when you lack B vitamins; for instance, cracks or crow's feet around the corners of your mouth are telltale signs of a deficiency of one or more. Another sign is memory loss.

B vitamins are also one of the best hangover prevention remedies for they help metabolize alcohol and reduce mental and oxidative stress while improving mental health; at their least, they can make hangovers shorter and less severe.

Breaking Down the B Vitamins

In the early 1900s, scientists discovered similar compounds they named a B vitamin, which eventually led to the eight essential B vitamins or the vitamin B complex: B1 thiamin (RDA 1.2 mg), B2 riboflavin (RDA 1.3 mg), B3 niacin (RDA 16 mg), B5 pantothenic acid (RDA 5 mg), B6 pyridoxine (RDA 1.7 mg), B7 biotin (RDA 30 mcg), B9 folic (RDA 400 mcg), and B12 cobalamin (RDA 2.4 mcg). Plus, they are three non-essential B vitamins (since your body can synthesize them): choline (RDA 550 mg), inositol (No RDA), para-aminobenzoic acid or PABA (No RDA).

Essentially all B vitamins are coenzymes needed to carry out many enzyme-related functions, from digesting or breaking down carbohydrates, fats, and proteins into glucose (energy) to maintaining healthy skin, hair, eyesight, muscle tone, nervous system, and brain. They also protect against chronic diseases by supporting a healthy immune system.

In addition, B1 thiamin, B2 riboflavin, B3 niacin, B5 pantothenic acid, B6 pyridoxine, B9 folate, and B12 cobalamin also help relieve stress and depression by synthesizing your mood-enhancing neurotransmitters, including dopamine and serotonin. Plus, B2 riboflavin also acts as an antioxidant and a coenzyme needed to increase your glutathione levels.

B6 pyridoxine, B9 folic, and B12 cobalamin are also needed to reduce levels of the non-essential amino acid homocysteine, which is known to damage the endothelial cells that line the interior surface of the blood vessels, increasing your risk of atherosclerosis, cardiovascular diseases, and dementia. So if you have high homocysteine levels (which ironically is also linked to depression by causing a neurotransmitter deficiency) you most likely lack these B vitamins.

But since all B vitamins work together (or why scientists call them a complex vitamin), the "inter-related functions of the eight B-vitamins and marshals evidence suggesting that adequate levels of all members of this group of micronutrients are essential for optimal physiological and neurological functioning," according to the review, B

Vitamins and the Brain: Mechanisms, Dose and Efficacy—A Review.

In other words, for overall better mental and physical health, take a vitamin B complex. Nevertheless, taking too much of one B vitamin can cause deficiencies in the others. Symptoms of a vitamin B deficiency include poor appetite, digestive problems, fatigue, headaches, memory loss, depression, nervousness, anxiety, poor coordination, muscle cramps, hair loss, and skin disorders.

A quick way to tell if you have a B vitamin deficiency is to look in the mirror and check out your mouth and tongue. If you are in a severe deficiency state, you'll have tiny cracks around your mouth and lips. And if your tongue is coated white (e.g., via alcohol dehydration) instead of its normal pink, there's a good chance you're low.

A Vitamin B Complex Renewal Plan

Your body can't synthesize (make) the eight essential B vitamins, so everyone needs a daily plan to renew them. And as with all vitamins, it's best to get your B vitamins from your diet. Although to get a healthy balance of all the B vitamins you need to consume a variety of foods such as whole grains, beans, nuts, seeds, avocados, bananas, green leafy vegetables, broccoli, spinach, lean meat, poultry, seafood, and eggs. Another option is to take a few tablespoons of Brewer's yeast, which is only lacking vitamin B12 (see Tip 47 - Brewer's Yeast: A Complete Meal).

And since vegetarians don't eat meat, a primary source of vitamin B12 (required to build red blood cells), they're at a higher risk of a B12 deficiency. An option for them is to take a B12 sublingual (Latin for "under the tongue") supplement.

If you take a multivitamin, it should already contain a vitamin B complex. But if you drink often, it's advised to also take a B complex supplement such as a "vitamin B complex 50 mg" that contains the eight essential and three non-essential B vitamins. And since B vitamins are water-soluble, there's a low risk of overdosing, your body usually uses what it needs and then pees (yellow) out the rest. To prevent spoilage (oxidation), store your vitamin B complex (and all vitamins) in a cool place with the lid tightly secured.

How are your B vitamins doing today? Check out your tongue as a reminder. If it's coated white, it might be time to stock up.

Tip 31

Health Benefits of Raw Nuts and Seeds

Raw nuts and seeds supply you with essential nutrients that naturally increase and sustain your energy levels while nourishing and protecting your cells against aging and disease.

They are some of the most nutrient-dense foods on earth. For instance, almonds, pecans, peanuts, walnuts, cashews, hazelnuts, pistachios, Brazil nuts, sunflower seeds, pumpkin seeds, and flaxseeds contain amino acids, B vitamins, vitamin E, fiber, calcium, magnesium, potassium, copper, zinc, selenium, iron, and polyunsaturated fats (omega-3 fatty acids), the heart and brain healthy fats that decrease bad LDL cholesterol and increase good HDL cholesterol.

They are also rich in antioxidants that guard against free radicals and oxidative stress.

And they all contain enzymes, the proteins known as the spark plugs of life needed to ignite and maintain vitality. So again, eat less overcooked or dead foods and more raw or live enzyme-containing foods with each meal to hold on to your youth.

Heart Food

"A greater consumption of tree nuts [walnuts] and peanuts is associated with a reduced risk of CVD mortality, as well as lower CVD events," according to the review, Nuts and Cardiovascular Disease [CVD] Prevention. Researchers also find the "risk factors associated with the development of CVD such as dyslipidemia [high LDL cholesterol], impaired vascular [blood vessel] function, and hypertension are improved with regular tree nut and peanut consumption through a range of mechanism associated with their nutrient-rich profiles."

"These findings suggest that nut consumption or factors associated with this nutritional behaviour may play a role in reducing the risk of atrial fibrillation [irregular heartbeat] and possibly heart failure," according to the study, Nut Consumption and Incidence of Seven Cardiovascular Disease. Researchers found that "Nut consumption ≥3 times/week was associated with an 18% reduced risk of atrial fibrillation."

Brain Food

Adults who consume 10 grams (two teaspoons) or more of nuts a day are "40% less likely to have poor cognitive function," according to the study, A Prospective Association of Nut Consumption with Cognitive Function in Chinese Adults Aged 55+, which included "4822 adults aged 55 and over participating in the China Health Nutrition Survey during 1991-2006." The participants mainly consumed peanuts.

Nuts are also "preventive agents against brain atrophy [deterioration] and memory loss," according to the review, Almond, Hazelnut and Walnut, Three Nuts for Neuroprotection in Alzheimer's Disease: A Neuropharmacological

Review of Their Bioactive Constituents. Researchers found them to "provide macronutrients, micronutrients, and phytochemicals [antioxidants] which affect several pathways in AD pathogenesis."

Although the walnut is most recognized for brain health since it ironically resembles the shape of the human brain. For instance, researchers "review evidence that early intervention with a walnut-enriched diet can reduce the risk and/or delay the onset or slow the progression of cognitive decline and dementia because of the elevated oxidative stress and inflammation involved in the aging process and dementia and the antioxidant and anti-inflammatory components of walnuts…[and found] substantial evidence from animal and human studies suggests that dietary consumption of walnuts (1–2 oz per day) can improve cognitive function and also reduce the risk of other diseases, such as cardiovascular disease, depression, and type 2 diabetes, which are risk factors for the development of dementia," according to the review, Beneficial Effects of Walnuts on Cognition and Brain Health.

And if you are pregnant, consuming a variety of nuts can help ensure your child has a healthy brain, according to the study, Maternal Nut Intake in Pregnancy and Child Neuropsychological Development Up to 8 Years Old: A Population-Based Cohort Study in Spain. Researchers "included 2208 mother-child pairs" and found that the children of mothers who consumed almonds, walnuts, pine nuts, peanuts, and hazelnuts during their first trimester scored higher on cognitive and memory tests.

Weight Control Food

Research has found that "a handful of nuts [1 ounce or 1/4 cup] daily is beneficial for the prevention of obesity and T2D [type 2 diabetes] because they are good sources of unsaturated fats, vegetable proteins, plant sterols, fiber, and antioxidants," according to the study, Long-Term Associations of Nut Consumption With Body Weight and Obesity. And they're "beneficial for weight control by contributing to satiety [the state of being full] and potentially improving long-term adherence to healthful diets."

Achieving a Complete Source of Protein

All nuts and seeds, however, lack one or more of the nine essential amino acids required to be a complete source of protein, but consuming a few together will do the trick. Take your pick from amino acid-rich almonds, walnuts, pecans, cashews, peanuts, hazelnuts, pistachios, Brazil nuts, sunflower seeds, pumpkin seeds, flaxseeds, chia seeds, and hemp seeds.

Why Raw Instead of Roasted?

Raw nuts and seeds have all their nutrients intact. But when roasted, it destroys their enzymes and decreases their vitamin and mineral levels. Roasting them also forms the chemical acrylamide linked to nerve damage and cancer.

So before purchasing packaged or bulk nuts and seeds, make sure the label states they are raw (and salt-free). And since most nuts and seeds contain pesticides, when possible, buy organic. Also look for nuts and seeds that are sprouted for they contain fewer anti-nutrients.

Removing Anti-Nutrients

Raw nuts and seeds, however, also contain anti-nutrients such as enzyme inhibitors and phytates that can lead to nutrient deficiencies and indigestion problems. To reduce their levels, the solution is to soak them in spring or distilled water with a tablespoon of salt for seven to eight hours. The other option is to sprout them in water, which usually takes longer. Either way, afterward, rinse them in a colander, dry with a paper towel, and refrigerate in an airtight container to prevent oxidation. And besides being easier to digest, soaking or sprouting nuts and seeds make them even more nutritious.

Health Goal

In 2003, the FDA approved the following qualified health claim for almonds, hazelnuts, peanuts, pecans, pistachios, and walnuts: "Scientific evidence suggests but does not prove that eating 1.5 ounces [1/3 cup] per day of most nuts, as part of a diet low in saturated fat and cholesterol, may reduce the risk of heart disease."

Nuts and seeds are also good sources of the amino acid tryptophan that improves your mood by boosting serotonin levels. Ideally, consume around a handful a day. And to make them sweeter and more nutritious, add some iron-rich raisins.

Tip 32

Scoring the Best Bread

Research finds that about half of Americans are still unsure what is the best bread to buy. Others now realize that Wonder Bread, the 1930s bread that became famous by its ad campaign: "The greatest thing since sliced bread" is not that wonderful since it's primarily made from chemically bleached white flour, making it significantly less healthier than whole wheat bread.

Studies find that consuming whole wheat bread reduces your risk of cardiovascular diseases, respiratory diseases, infectious diseases, liver diseases, diabetes, colon cancer, and mortality. To make whole wheat bread they use the entire whole wheat kernel or wheat berry: the bran (outer layer), which includes insoluble fiber, protein, B vitamins, iron, and antioxidants; the germ (embryo), which includes essential fatty acids (omega-3 fatty acids), antioxidants, protein, B vitamins, vitamin E, and zinc; and the endosperm (starchy interior layer), which includes carbohydrates, soluble fiber, protein, B vitamins, and iron. Then, after nature's maturing process, all three layers are ground, mixed, and made into whole wheat bread.

On the contrary, to make white bleached bread (flour) they use just the endosperm by milling the wheat berries to remove the bran and germ (for a longer shelf life). Then they skip nature's roughly one month maturing process and instead use bleaching (maturing) agents that only take a few days. And some conventional farmers still use the herbicide (weedkiller) glyphosate to speed up the harvesting of their grain crops via a process called crop desiccation (the removal of moisture): a few weeks before harvest, farmers spray glyphosate (Roundup) to kill the plant so the crop dries out faster. So except for organic bread, almost all other breads (even labeled non-GMO) may still contain some glyphosate. Though, under public pressure, some farms are banning chemical desiccation.

Milling flour white also reduces nutrients, so it must be enriched with at least vitamin B1 thiamin, B2 riboflavin, B3 niacin, and some iron, according to FDA regulations. The FDA also requires bread made from this flour to be labeled "enriched," or a telltale sign that at least some of its flour may be bleached.

The most widely used flour bleaching agent is chlorine dioxide gas, which accelerates the flour's aging process via oxidation. But it also creates a toxic byproduct called alloxan that has been found in trace amounts in some bleached flours. Alloxan generates deadly reactive oxygen species (ROS free radicals) that destroy pancreatic beta cells required for producing insulin, the key hormone that opens the doors of your cells to let glucose or energy in. Therefore, researchers use alloxan to induce diabetes, a.k.a. impaired insulin production, in laboratory animals. So there's an obvious connection between consuming bleached flour and diabetes. Though if you have an insulin problem, the mineral chromium increases its production.

Consuming bleached white bread also spikes your blood glucose levels, causing a potential insulin or diabetic problem. The Glycemic Index (GI) assigns food a number from 0 to 100 that represents the rise in glucose levels a few hours after consumption, known as the food's glycemic (sugar) load. And it uses white bread as a reference food!

Again, foods that ranks high on the GI also means they are low in fiber. For instance, a slice of white bread contains only around 0.5 grams of fiber, whereas a slice of whole wheat bread contains around 2 grams; mixed whole grains 4 grams. So when you consume whole wheat bread (or high-fiber complex carbohydrates) you'll experience healthier bowel movements. But when you consume white bread (or low-fiber refined carbohydrates) you're more likely to experience constipation (and a higher risk of diabetes).

It's also harder to lose weight if you regularly consume white bread. Your liver converts extra carbohydrates into triglycerides (fats), especially from sweets and (refined) white bread. According to a Tufts University study, people who mainly consume white bread (which is widely used in processed and fast foods) have larger waistlines than whole wheat consumers. And a Mediterranean cohort study of 9,267 Spanish university graduates also found that "Consumption of white bread (≥2 portions/day) showed a significant direct association with the risk of becoming overweight/obese."

Many countries have banned bleaching flour, and in the USA, food labels must state that its flour is bleached.

Also Avoid Bromated Flour

Also avoid bread containing bromated flour or potassium bromate, a food additive linked to thyroid disorders and cancer. It's mainly used in large-scale baking operations for it strengthens the dough and gives it more elasticity and rise. Hence, it's also found in many processed and fast foods.

Bromated flour is banned in some countries. In the US, however, only bread and other bakery goods sold in California are required to have a label warning stating that it contains the carcinogen potassium bromate.

Reading Bread Labels: Scoring the Best Bread

Fortunately, it's easy to tell what a loaf of bread is mainly made from because FDA regulations require food (and beverage) ingredients to be listed by weight, or whatever weighs the most is listed first, and so forth. So for a healthier loaf of bread, avoid breads that first list white flour, bleached white flour, enriched bleached white flour, bleached wheat flour, or enriched bleached wheat flour.

Instead, the better options are to buy bread that first lists whole wheat flour or unbleached flour. Though just make sure the bread doesn't also contain sugar, artificial sweeteners, high fructose corn syrup, canola oil, soybean oil, and artificial preservatives.

Even better, just buy organic whole wheat bread. By USDA organic regulations, it cannot contain bleached flour, bromated flour, glyphosate, artificial sweeteners, high fructose corn syrup, and artificial preservatives. The first ingredient on an organic wheat bread usually states it contains organic sprouted (live) whole wheat berries, organic whole wheat, or organic whole grains. Also look for flourless.

And similar to fruits and vegetables, whole wheat bread

ranks high in antioxidants. A few slices a day is ideal.

Tip 33

Wheatgrass Juice "Healing" Shots

The health benefits of consuming wheatgrass have been renowned for over 5,000 years. Resembling a typical blade of green grass, it grows from the sprouted seeds of wheat berries, used to make whole wheat bread.

And when juiced, it becomes a concentrated source of nutrition. For instance, a "1 ounce [shot] of wheatgrass juice is equivalent in vitamins, minerals and amino acids found in 1 Kg [2.2 pounds] of green leafy vegetables," according to the review, Health and Nutritional Benefits of Wheat Grass Juice. Anyhow, it's a potent shot of healing.

Its healing properties are found in its unique balance of amino acids, chlorophyll, enzymes, antioxidants, vitamin A, B vitamins, vitamin C, vitamin D, vitamin E, vitamin K, and the minerals calcium, magnesium, manganese, iron, phosphorus, chromium, selenium, copper, and zinc.

Among its many health benefits, research finds wheatgrass "to help diminish fatigue, improve sleep, increase strength, naturally regulate blood pressure and blood sugar, support weight loss, improve digestion and elimination, support healthy skin, teeth, eyes, muscles, and joints, improve the function of our heart-lungs and reproductive organs, heal ulcers and skin sores, slow cellular aging, improve mental function, and is beneficial in arthritis and muscle cramping, thalassemia, hemolytic anemia, cancer, asthma, allergy, inflammatory bowel disease, and detoxification," according to the study, A Pilot Study on Wheatgrass Juice for its Phytochemical [Antioxidant], Nutritional and Therapeutic Potential on Chronic Diseases.

Wheatgrass a.k.a. Green Blood

Wheatgrass is recognized as containing one of the highest concentrations of chlorophyll (over 70%), which is why it's called "Green Blood."

Chlorophyll, the green plant pigment that achieves photosynthesis needed for generating oxygen, is also structurally similar to hemoglobin (heme for iron and globin for protein), the iron-rich protein found in your red blood cells that transports oxygen throughout your body. The main difference is that hemoglobin has iron as its central atom, and chlorophyll has magnesium. Either way, the results are healthier red blood cells and more oxygen.

Chlorophyll also contains powerful antioxidant and chelation properties that cleanse your blood, lymph system, liver, kidneys, pancreas, colon, and lungs of toxins and heavy metals. Research finds it also prevents oxidative stress as well as glutathione, the master antioxidant.

Other greens high in chlorophyll include broccoli, Brussels sprouts, kale, spinach, parsley, romaine lettuce, green bell peppers, green beans, green peas, collard greens, turnip greens, and watercress.

Finding a Wheatgrass Shot

A shot of wheatgrass costs around $4 at a juice bar. The other option is to juice at home by either growing your own wheatgrass or purchasing a bag of pre-cut wheatgrass. You'll also need a wheatgrass juicer or a cold press juicer because the standard centrifugal vegetable juicer with its high rpm motor cannot break down fine grasses—they zoom right through it. (But not all cold press juicers juice wheatgrass.)

Health Goal

Drinking a shot of wheatgrass a few times a week can help make a world of difference in your health. And like other shots, they're felt instantly. Although signs of it working include improved breathing and increased energy levels.

Wheatgrass is also an effective hangover remedy by supplying your body and mind with a shot of fresh oxygen.

Tip 34

Organic Produce or Bust?

Are you still sitting on the fence regarding buying organic fruits and vegetables? After all, aren't they all healthy for me?

A main health concern with consuming conventional or non-organic produce is that many are sprayed with not just one but a variety of chemical pesticides needed to ward off a variety of pests. So when you consume a non-organic fruit or vegetable, you are also most likely consuming not just one, but a variety of harmful pesticides. For instance, "One sample of mustard greens had 20 different pesticides, and some kale and collard samples had as many as 17," according to the Environmental Working Group's 2021 Shopper's Guide to Pesticides in Produce.

Consequently, the blood and urine of those who mainly consume non-organic produce contains a "cocktail" of pesticide residues, according to the CDC. And it's impossible to completely wash-off pesticides because the plant has absorbed them throughout its growth cycle; therefore, they are embedded in the plant's cell walls.

On the contrary, organic farmers control pests with natural enemies such as parasitoid wasps, hover flies, damsel bugs, and ladybugs.

Health Concerns with Ingesting Pesticides

The "numerous negative health effects that have been associated with chemical pesticides include, among other effects, dermatological, gastrointestinal, neurological, carcinogenic, respiratory, reproductive, and endocrine effects," according to the review, Chemical Pesticides and Human Health: The Urgent Need for a New Concept in Agriculture via researchers from the National and Kapodistrian University of Athens, Greece.

And men who regularly consume non-organic fruits and vegetables high in pesticides reduced their sperm count by 49%, according to the Harvard University study, Fruit and Vegetable Intake and Their Pesticide Residues in Relation to Semen Quality Among Men From a Fertility Clinic.

Whereas women who regularly consume non-organic fruits and vegetables high in pesticides reduced their chances of becoming pregnant by 18%, according to an another Harvard University study, Association Between Pesticide Residue Intake From Consumption of Fruits and Vegetables and Pregnancy Outcomes Among Women Undergoing Infertility Treatment With Assisted Reproductive Technology.

And these findings "suggest that an offspring's risk of autism spectrum disorder increases following prenatal exposure to ambient [surrounding] pesticides," according to the study, Prenatal and Infant Exposure to Ambient Pesticides and Autism Spectrum Disorder in Children: Population Based Case-Control Study, which included 2961 individuals diagnosed with autism.

Plus, parents should beware that organophosphate pesticides (OP), which are routinely sprayed on many non-organic fruits and vegetables, also increases a child's risk of attention deficit hyperactivity disorder (ADHD), according to the review, Increased Risk of ADHD Associated With Early Exposure to Pesticides, PCBs [Polychlorinated Biphenyls]. The research "found that even children who experience more typical levels of pesticide exposure, such as from eating pesticide-treated fruits and vegetables, have a higher risk of developing the disorder."

Health Benefits of Going Organic

Switching to organic produce for only six days can reduce your pesticide levels by 60%, according to the study, Organic Diet Intervention Significantly Reduces Urinary Pesticide Levels in US Children and Adults. Researchers "observed significant reductions in urinary levels of thirteen pesticide metabolites and parent compounds representing OP, neonicotinoid, and pyrethroid insecticides and the herbicide 2, 4-D following the introduction of an organic diet." Likewise, a follow-up study showed a 70% reduction of the herbicide glyphosate in six days.

Going organic also reduces your risk of cancer, according to the study, Association of Frequency of Organic Food Consumption With Cancer Risk. Researchers found that "In a population-based cohort study of 68,946 French adults, a significant [25%] reduction in the risk of cancer was observed among high consumers of organic." It reduced their risk of lymphoma (non-Hodgkin's), skin, prostate, colorectal, and breast cancer, which is supported by the study, Association Between Organic Food Consumption and Breast Cancer Risk: Findings from the Sister Study (P18-038-19). Researchers here "used data from 39,563 Sister Study participants aged 35 to 74 years…[and found that] organic produce consumption was associated with reduced breast cancer risk."

Regarding nutrients, research finds that "Organic crops contained significantly more vitamin C, iron, magnesium, and phosphorus and significantly less nitrates than conventional crops," according to the study, Nutritional Quality of Organic Versus Conventional Fruits, Vegetables, and Grains.

Organic crops also contain between 18% to 69% more antioxidants than non-organic crops, according to the study, Higher Antioxidant and Lower Cadmium Concentrations and Lower Incidence of Pesticide Residues in Organically Grown Crops: A Systematic Literature Review and Meta-Analyses, which included 343 peer-reviewed publications. Researchers found that since organic crops are grown without chemical fertilizers and pesticides, organic grapes, for instance, contain more anthocyanin antioxidants, organic apples more quercetin antioxidants, tomatoes more lycopene antioxidants, and so forth.

How to Know It's Real Organic

Look for bags of produce that contain the USDA Organic Seal, which means they cannot contain non-organic fertilizers, pesticides, herbicides, insecticides, fungicides, and GMOs.

When buying loose produce, look for its small PLU (price look-up) code sticker. Organic produce has a five-digit code starting with 9, non-organic produce has a four-digit code starting with 3 or 4, and GMO produce (apples, corn, summer squash, white potatoes, papayas, alfalfa, soybeans, sugar beets, and pink pineapples) has a five-digit code starting with 8.

The Main Produce to Buy Organic

According to the USDA's Pesticide Data Program (PDP), the produce with the highest levels of pesticides, or what you should always buy organic, include apples, peaches, nectarines, blueberries, cherries, strawberries, grapes, pears, kiwi, lettuce, celery, spinach, tomatoes, white potatoes, winter squash, green beans, kale, cucumbers, bell peppers, and hot peppers.

The produce with the lowest levels of pesticides, or what you don't always have to buy organic, include avocados, bananas, lemons, mangos, pineapples, papayas, cantaloupes, honeydew melons, eggplants, mushrooms, asparagus, broccoli, Brussels sprouts, cabbage, cauliflower, sweet potatoes, sweet peas, sweet corn, carrots, onions, and garlic.

For the latest information on pesticides in produce (based on the USDA PDP), see the Environmental Working Group's Annual Dirty Dozen and Clean Fifteen Shopper's Guide.

Also Buy Organic Packaged Foods

When possible, also buy organic packaged foods to avoid the more than 2,000 potentially toxic FDA allowed additives in conventional packaged foods, including chemical preservatives, flavors, and colors.

But fewer than 40 synthetic ingredients are permitted in organic packaged foods. And before approval, the USDA Organic Standards Board must first confirm they are safe for humans and the environment.

The Cost of Going Organic

The cost of organic produce averages 15% to 25% higher than conventional produce. Although the cost is coming down because more farms are switching to organic: it also protects the planet from climate change by sequestering carbon back into the soil. So if the organic movement continues, then one day, the price of organic produce will match the price of conventional produce, which you can now find at some stores (e.g., Trader Joe's) and on sale.

Tip 35

Cruciferous Vegetables for Cancer Prevention and Overall Better Health

People who regularly consume cruciferous vegetables such as broccoli, kale, Brussels sprouts, cauliflower, and cabbage reduce their risk of cancer by 64%, according to the review, Brassica [Cruciferous] Vegetables and Cancer Prevention, the results of six cohort studies and 74 case-control studies. Many other studies have found similar results.

So what do cruciferous vegetables have over other foods in cancer prevention? They contain high amounts of glucosinolates, the plant's bitter-tasting sulfur compounds that defend it against pests. Studies find they also defend human cells against carcinogens by activating and increasing the body's cellular defense antioxidants, including glutathione, superoxide dismutase, and catalase.

Glucosinolates are released by the plant's defense enzyme, myrosinase, after they are cut, chopped, or chewed. This reaction then forms potent sulfur compounds called isothiocyanates (e.g., sulforaphane) and indole-3-carbinol, which are attributed to the main health benefits of consuming glucosinolates.

The sulfur compound sulforaphane, for instance, is a powerful anticarcinogen and antioxidant that lowers your risk of esophageal, bladder, prostate, breast, stomach, colon, and lung cancer.

Sulforaphane also helps guard against Alzheimer's disease by protecting brain cells from free radicals and oxidative stress. It also helps restore the glutamate amino acid imbalance linked to schizophrenia by increasing glutathione levels.

If you are in an occupation that could cause head injuries, such as a quarterback, research shows that sulforaphane strengthens and protects the network of capillaries known as the blood-brain barrier (BBB), making you more resilient to head injuries.

The other sulfur compound, indole-3-carbinol, also acts as a powerful anticarcinogen and antioxidant that lowers your risk of rectal, cervical, prostate, breast, colon, and lung cancer. It also reduces levels of inflammation and unhealthy fats, lowering your risk of cardiovascular disease, obesity, diabetes, and fatty liver disease.

Indole-3-carbinol may also be the key to inhibiting the herpes simplex virus. For example, an in vitro (test tube) study on human and monkey cells found it to block the herpes virus from reproducing by 99.9%!

These powerful sulfur compounds are also found in other members of the cruciferous family of vegetables, such as arugula, bok choy, rutabaga, watercress, and collard greens.

In addition, cruciferous vegetables are also a good source of plant protein, vitamin A, vitamin C, vitamin E, folate, calcium, magnesium, potassium, fiber, and other antioxidants such as alpha lipoic acid and CoQ10, which are also needed for energy production.

Mental Health

Cruciferous vegetables also contain tryptophan, the amino acid that helps overcome depression by producing serotonin. They're also a good source of the antioxidants lutein and zeaxanthin that not only protect your eyes from oxidative stress but also your brain while improving your working memory or recall.

And their sulfur compounds also contain chelating properties that help detoxify heavy metals (e.g., aluminum, arsenic, cadmium, mercury, and lead) before they can lodge in your brain and cause neurological disorders.

Lung Health

Research finds that the "intake of individual cruciferous vegetables, especially consumed as raw, were significantly associated with reduction of lung cancer risk," according to the study, Cruciferous Vegetable Intake is Inversely Associated With Lung Cancer Risk Among Smokers: A Case-Control Study. "Our findings are consistent with the smoking-related carcinogen-modulating effect of isothiocyanates, a group of phytochemicals [plant chemicals] uniquely present in cruciferous vegetables."

Furthermore, a Chinese meta-analysis found that cruciferous vegetables reduced lung cancer risk in women. Researchers here found that isothiocyanates are a key to inhibiting tumorigenesis.

Bone Health

Cruciferous vegetables also help build and maintain strong bones by providing them with a good source of calcium and vitamin C, which helps to improve calcium absorption. A cup of kale, for instance, contains around 90 mg of calcium and 80 mg of vitamin C, and a cup of raw broccoli 45 mg of calcium and 80 mg of vitamin C. The RDA for calcium is around 1000 mg and 90 mg for vitamin C.

Protection Against Eating Red Meat

Studies find that people who regularly consume red meat have a higher risk of stomach and colon cancer; however, those who also regularly consume cruciferous vegetables reduced their risk. So have some kale or broccoli with your next steak.

Best to Consume Cruciferous Vegetables Raw or Lightly Steamed

Overcooking cruciferous vegetables significantly reduces their amounts of vitamins, minerals, antioxidants, enzymes, and glucosinolates.

For example, the "bioavailability of ITCs [isothiocyanates] from fresh [raw] broccoli is approximately three times greater than that from cooked broccoli, in which myrosinase [enzyme] is inactivated," according to the study, Disposition of Glucosinolates and Sulforaphane in Humans After Ingestion of Steamed and Fresh Broccoli. Or, for instance, when you over steam broccoli to where it turns a darker shade of green, you have just inactivated the enzyme myrosinase, needed to release its glucosinolates.

Steaming them is the next best option. Research has found that "steaming [for 5 min.] led to the lowest loss of total indole glucosinolates (36.8%), while stir-frying [5 min.] and stir-frying [2 min.]/boiling [3 min.] presented the highest (67% and 64%, respectively)," according to the study, Effects of Different Cooking Methods on Health-Promoting Compounds of Broccoli. So it's best to steam them for 3 to 5 minutes or when broccoli turns a lighter shade of green.

But avoid microwaving cruciferous (and all) vegetables. Research has found "clear disadvantages were detected when cooking in a microwave due to the high loss of vitamin C (40%) and total glucosinolates (74%)," according to the study, Glucosinolates and Vitamin C Content in Edible Parts of Broccoli Florets After Domestic Cooking. "Therefore, we can conclude that a large quantity of glucosinolates and vitamin C will be consumed in steamed broccoli when compared to the other cooking processes."

Yet another broccoli study found that microwaving destroyed 97% of its flavonoid antioxidants. Hence, the "consumption of microwaved foods resulted in a significant decrease in antioxidant protection and may be implicated in the pathogenesis oxidative stress and degenerative diseases," according to the study, Effect of Ingestion of Microwaved Foods on Serum Anti-oxidant Enzymes and Vitamins of Albino Rats.

Although it's not recommended to consume cruciferous vegetables with every meal because they also contain goitrogen compounds (thioglycosides) that can inhibit your iodine uptake needed for a healthy thyroid gland. If you have a thyroid issue, steaming them will reduce their levels.

For cancer prevention and overall better health, consume one or two servings (cups) a day, raw or lightly steamed.

Tip 36

Lemon Aid

Drinking a glass of freshly squeezed lemon in spring water is one of the best all-around health drinks.

Lemons contain organic water, enzymes, calcium, magnesium, potassium, iron, B vitamins, vitamin C, citric acid, and citrus flavonoid antioxidants, which guard "against oxidative stress, inflammation, diabetes, dyslipidemia, endothelial dysfunction, and atherosclerosis," according to the review, Beneficial Effects of Citrus Flavonoids on Cardiovascular and Metabolic Health. Lemons also contain limonoid antioxidants that are mainly found in their seeds and peel (inner white skin). And as with flavonoid antioxidants, limonoids also increase your glutathione levels.

An easy way to grasp the power of antioxidants is to squeeze lemon juice on a slice of apple. Normally, it would turn brown in a short time due to oxidation (free radicals), but with lemon's antioxidants, the apple takes significantly longer to turn brown.

Natural Source of Citric Acid

Lemons are a great source of citric acid, which naturally increases your energy levels and improves nutrient absorption. It's also a potent antioxidant that protects your liver against free radicals and oxidative stress. And it contains antimicrobial properties that help prevent bacterial and fungal infections. It's more known, however, as a remedy for kidney stones (calcium oxalate stones) by increasing your urinary levels of citrate (an ester of citric acid), which prevents stone formation. It also helps prevent gout by reducing uric acid levels.

Besides lemons, citrus acid is also found in limes, oranges, grapefruits, and tangerines. But it's not to be confused with the manufactured form of citrus acid, a food additive made from the Aspergillus niger fungus that's added to many packaged foods and beverages to prevent spoilage by increasing pH acidity levels. Since 1919, almost all the world's citrus acid production has been made from this fungus, which is also well-known for causing black mold on fruits and vegetables. Research also finds that it significantly increases inflammation in humans. And it's linked to causing oxidative stress damage to mice livers. Still, the FDA deems it safe.

Liver Aid

Lemons help maintain a healthy liver by flushing out toxins and providing it with essential vitamins, minerals, enzymes, and antioxidants.

Research has also "showed that lemon juice might be a potential dietary supplement for the prevention and treatment of liver injury related to chronic alcohol consumption," according to the study, the Protective Effects of Lemon Juice on Alcohol-Induced Liver Injury in Mice. "Treatment with lemon juice reduced the level of lipid peroxidation to a normal level, which showed a significant protective effect of lemon juice against alcohol-induced oxidative stress." So add a lemon wedge to your next drink.

Smoker's Aid

Lemon's citrus acid and other antioxidants help detoxify the body from the many carcinogens (free radicals) found in tobacco smoke, such as benzene, cadmium, tar, arsenic, formaldehyde, and lead. So have a lemon and water with your next smoke.

Weight-Loss Aid

Citric acid helps to burn extra pounds by breaking down fat molecules. And lemon's antioxidants have shown to suppress obesity in mice fed a high-fat diet. So also have a lemon and water with your next fatty meal.

Indigestion and Heartburn Aid

There is a misconception about lemons: that they only create an acidic reaction in the body. But once metabolized, research finds its alkaline minerals calcium, magnesium, and potassium reduce its citric acid levels to eventually create an alkaline reaction, which helps prevent bloating, gas, indigestion, and heartburn. Plus, its digestive enzymes also help relieve these conditions.

There is, of course, a limit to consuming any acid-containing food since too much can cause indigestion and heartburn. For most, a lemon a day is ideal.

Preparing

Before slicing a lemon, wash it well to remove any harmful bacteria that could transmit from the outside to the inside. Then cut a quarter wedge and squeeze it into a glass of spring water. Stir well.

Although citrus acid can harm your tooth enamel (though a little can help prevent tooth decay by killing bacteria). The solution is to swallow it without allowing the lemon juice to wash over your teeth or just drink it out of a paper straw.

Try to drink a few glasses a day, especially when you need a quick pick-me-up to beat stress, depression, or a hangover. And to maximize its health benefits, add some of the lemon's inner white skin. Also inhaling the scent of fresh lemon helps relieve stress.

A lemon a day keeps the doctor away.

Tip 37

Tea Break

After water, tea is the most widely consumed drink in the world. It contains some impressive health properties that naturally increase your energy levels while helping to preserve a healthy mind and body.

At the heart of it, tea drinkers live longer because they have a healthier cardiovascular system. According to the study, Tea Consumption and the Risk of Atherosclerotic [Hardening of Arteries] Cardiovascular Disease and All-Cause Mortality: The China-PAR project, researchers studied the tea consumption habits of 100,902 Chinese adults and found that compared with never or non-habitual tea drinkers, habitual tea drinkers had a 39% lower risk of incident heart disease and stroke, a 56% lower risk of fatal heart disease and stroke, and a 29% lower risk of all-cause mortality.

Research also finds that regularly drinking tea improves your mental health by increasing brain structure connectivity or connections. It also "influences psychopathological symptoms (e.g., reduction of anxiety), cognition (e.g., benefits in memory and attention) and brain function (e.g., activation of working memory seen in functional MRI)," according to the review, Green Tea Effects on Cognition, Mood and Human Brain Function: A Systematic Review.

Drinking tea also reduces your risk of dementia. And

recent in vitro (lab) research finds that tea prevents brain amyloid plaques from forming and breaks up existing plaques and neurofibrillary tangles, the two leading causes of Alzheimer's disease. Tea also protects brain cells from free radicals and oxidative stress while promoting hippocampal (hippocampus) neurogenesis.

All Teas Are Healthy

Even though most studies have focused on the health benefits of drinking green tea, all tea leaves come from the same tea plant called Camellia sinensis. So whether it's green, white, oolong, or black tea, they're all healthy for they contain powerful anti-inflammatory properties and antioxidants that also increase blood levels of your internal antioxidants glutathione, superoxide dismutase, and catalase.

Tea's medicinal (healing) benefits date to around 2800 BCE. Since then, "The evidence supporting the health benefits of tea drinking grows stronger with each new study that is published in the scientific literature," according to the paper, Tea and Health: Studies in Humans. For instance, "Various studies suggest that polyphenolic compounds present in green and black tea are associated with beneficial effects in prevention of cardiovascular diseases, particularly of atherosclerosis and coronary heart disease. In addition, anti-aging, antidiabetic and many other health beneficial effects associated with tea consumption."

We also now know that tea induces autophagy (Greek for self-eating), your body's natural way of removing damaged cellular components to regenerate healthier cells. Tea also helps keep your skin youthful by increasing collagen and elastin production while inhibiting the enzymes that break down these structural building proteins.

Green Tea Contains More Polyphenols (Antioxidants)

A tea leaf's quantity of polyphenols (plant defense compounds) depends on how the tea leaves are processed: the least oxidized (exposed to air and heat), the more polyphenols and antioxidants.

Therefore, green tea (and white tea) contains the highest amount of polyphenols because its leaves are the least oxidized, which is why their leaves retain their color. Whereas oolong tea leaves are partially oxidized or in the middle. And black tea leaves are fully oxidized, resulting in their dark green or black color.

Because green tea is the least oxidized, it contains a higher concentration of the powerful polyphenol epigallocatechin gallate (EGCG) than oolong and black tea. EGCG, a flavonoid polyphenol, is one of tea's most researched and abundant antioxidants. Among its many health benefits, it activates your immune system's T cells (white blood cells) to guard against infections and diseases. Research also finds that EGCG inhibits cancer formation by blocking an enzyme essential for cancer to grow and spread. It also boosts levels of p53, an anticancer protein that destroys cancerous cells and repairs DNA damage, a root cause of cancer.

It's also the main antioxidant that may protect your brain from developing Alzheimer's disease.

Lung Protection

Tea's EGCG also reduces cell DNA damage caused by tobacco smoke, according to the study, Effect of Increased Tea Consumption on Oxidative DNA Damage Among Smokers. Researchers "suggest that regular green tea drinking might protect smokers from oxidative damages and could reduce cancer risk or other diseases caused by free radicals associated with smoking."

And "Despite the high consumption of tobacco, Asia and Japan, in particular, have among the lowest incidences of arteriosclerosis and lung cancer per capital," according to the review, Green Tea, the "Asian Paradox," and Cardiovascular Disease. Why? They drink tea daily. So smokers should also drink tea.

Liver Protection

Research finds that tea's antioxidants help protect your liver cells against alcoholic fatty liver disease and non-alcoholic fatty liver disease caused by a poor diet.

Bone Protection

Research also finds that tea's anti-inflammatory properties and antioxidants help maintain strong bones while protecting against osteoporosis, the loss of bone density.

Other research found that combining stretching exercises with tea's antioxidant gallic acid decreases osteoarthritis inflammation and increases the production of cartilage proteins. So stretch with a cup of tea. Gallic acid is also found in berries, nuts, and wine.

Gut Health

Tea's polyphenols promote a healthy gut microbiota by increasing the growth and diversity of beneficial gut bacteria and inhibiting the growth of pathogenic bacteria.

Oral Health

Other research has found that tea's antioxidants protect against tooth decay, cavities, and periodontal disease. It also contains a natural source of fluoride and antibacterial properties that help reduce the buildup of tooth plaque.

Caffeine: Tea vs. Coffee

Per cup, tea contains less than half the caffeine found in coffee. Plus, tea contains the amino acid L-theanine that's well-known for producing a calming sense of relaxed awareness (unlike coffee's intense buzz) by increasing your mood-enhancing neurotransmitters dopamine, serotonin, and gamma-aminobutyric acid (GABA), the anti-anxiety neurotransmitter.

How to Obtain Tea's Maximum Health Benefits

To get the most health benefits out of a cup of tea, heat spring water to a gentle boil (tiny bubbles) and slowly pour it over a tea bag. Then let it steep for around two to four minutes. The problem with steeping with boiling water (and for too long) is that it burns the tea leaves, creating a strong bitter taste that may also cause an upset stomach if you drink it without food. Research also finds that drinking strong tea can hinder your iron absorption.

It's also recommended to drink organic teas because many non-organic teas are reported to contain high levels of pesticides, environmental pollutants, and heavy metals. Plus, research finds that over-boiling non-organic teas leach even more contaminants into the brew. And to prevent ingesting plastics, search for tea brands that use plastic-free tea bags.

One or two cups of organic tea a day is ideal, hot or iced. For a healthy sweetener, add a teaspoon of raw honey.

Tip 38

Coffee's Wake Up Concerns

Worldwide, around three billion cups of coffee are consumed daily. That makes coffee (or caffeine: pronounced ka-FEEN) the most widely used mind-altering drug in the world. An unfortunate side effect is that "clinical studies are showing that some caffeine users become dependent on the drug and are unable to reduce consumption despite knowledge of recurrent health problems associated with continued use," according to the review, Caffeine Use Disorder: A Comprehensive Review and Research Agenda.

Although many studies find that coffee is healthy because it contains antioxidants, including high amounts of chlorogenic acid, a powerful free radical scavenger. But research also finds that high intakes of chlorogenic acid raise your homocysteine levels, a predictor for oxidative stress and cardiovascular disease, according to the study, Consumption of High Doses of Chlorogenic Acid, Present in Coffee, or of Black Tea Increases Plasma Total Homocysteine Concentrations in Humans.

Plus, the high temperature required to roast coffee beans creates the chemical acrylamide, a probable human carcinogen.

Cardiovascular Concerns

Studies also find that drinking too much coffee increases blood pressure levels, potentially harming your blood vessels and heart muscle, which is a big concern for the hypertension-prone and those who currently have high blood pressure, the silent killer. The last thing they need is to consume anything that will artificially increase their heartbeat.

Furthermore, "We observed here that even moderate consumption of unfiltered coffee increases the amounts of proinflammatory markers of ischemic [lack of blood flow] heart disease," according to the study, Associations Between Coffee Consumption and Inflammatory Markers in Healthy Persons: The ATTICA Study.

Other studies find that unfiltered coffees such as French press and espressos contain high levels of cafestol, a molecule that elevates bad LDL cholesterol levels by suppressing the production of bile acid, needed to eliminate it from your body.

Stress Connection

Coffee's caffeine also stimulates your adrenal glands to release your stress hormones: adrenaline (epinephrine), norepinephrine, and cortisol. This results in the short-term benefits of heightened awareness and more energy. But, afterward, your body becomes overstimulated, resulting in lower energy levels. Either way, it's unhealthy for these stress hormones to run daily throughout your system, including increasing your risk of premature aging.

A caffeine-induced release of your stress hormones also raises your blood pressure levels, which over time can lead to heart disease, according to the study, Caffeine Affects Cardiovascular and Neuroendocrine Activation at Work and Home. Researchers found that "Repeated daily blood pressure elevations and increases in stress reactivity caused by caffeine consumption could contribute to an increased risk of coronary heart disease in the adult population."

Vitamins, Minerals, and Blood Sugar Concerns

Research finds that coffee reduces B vitamins, vitamin D, calcium, magnesium, potassium, zinc, and iron levels. Other research finds that drinking coffee on an empty stomach after a night of disturbed sleep skyrockets your blood sugar levels. Therefore, eat before drinking coffee to control blood sugar levels and take a multivitamin after drinking coffee to restore nutrient levels.

Tip 39

Melatonin Nightcap

Having trouble falling asleep on time? Are you concerned about the side effects of taking pharmaceutical sleep-aid drugs? You should be; just read the fine print.

The good news is that your body produces a natural nightcap, a hormone called melatonin. And since it comes out at night, it's nicknamed the "Dracula Hormone."

Your Sleep-Wake Cycle: The Circadian Rhythm

Melatonin's primary function is to regulate your body's sleep-wake cycle, known as the circadian rhythm. This is your 24-hour internal body clock that plays a critical role in when you fall asleep and rise.

Here's how the sleep-wake cycle is supposed to work: after sunset, your pineal gland, a pea-size light-sensitive organ in your brain, starts to release the sleep-inducing hormone melatonin into your bloodstream, which eventually builds up to a point to induce sleep. Then when morning comes, the pineal gland releases the mood-enhancing hormone serotonin. If all is working properly, the results are a better night's sleep and waking up feeling more alert and motivated.

But for some, their natural ability to produce normal

melatonin levels decrease with age, which may be linked to a history of consuming drinks high in caffeine (e.g., coffee, energy drinks) and foods high in table salt, refined sugars, and refined carbohydrates (e.g., fast foods, processed foods) for they disrupt the sleep-wake cycle.

Melatonin's Other Functions

While you're sleeping, melatonin provides other vital functions:

- It builds a strong immune system, increases muscle strength, and helps maintain a healthy weight.

- It acts as a potent antioxidant that guards your body against oxidative stress or uncontrolled free radicals.

- It helps prevent the growth of lung, colon, liver, pancreas, stomach, and breast cancer cells by helping to repair DNA damage.

- It reduces inflammation and helps to reverse the cell and organ damage caused by consuming foods high in triglycerides (fats) and LDL cholesterol. And it protects against strokes.

Boosting Melatonin Through Diet

Melatonin is available in supplements, but before going that route, at nighttime, consume foods that are sources of melatonin and the amino acid tryptophan, the precursor to producing melatonin. As the saying goes, eating turkey makes you sleepy because it contains tryptophan.

Sources of melatonin include eggs, corn, barley, oats, brown rice, walnuts, pistachios, tomatoes, red grapes, cherries, black cherry juice, olive oil, red wine, and beer. Sources of tryptophan include turkey, chicken, salmon, shrimp, eggs, milk, whole grains, brown rice, green peas, beans, peanuts, walnuts, pumpkin seeds, and Brewer's yeast.

Research finds, however, that a magnesium deficiency can decrease your melatonin levels. Magnesium-rich foods (similar to tryptophan-rich foods) to consume include salmon, whole grains, bran, brown rice, almonds, peanut butter, pumpkin seeds, peas, beans, and bananas.

A Corn and Pea Sleep Remedy

Since corn is a source of melatonin, and green peas a source of tryptophan, consuming a bowl of them can produce enough melatonin to induce a good night's sleep. And for an even healthier snack, hold the artery-clogging butter and add some artery-healthy extra virgin olive oil or lemon juice.

Melatonin Supplements

Melatonin supplements are known for helping to overcome insomnia and jet lag without the hazards or side effects of taking prescription drugs. For best results, keep the dosage low or between 0.3 to 3 mg. Research finds consuming higher doses can make your brain's melatonin receptors less responsive. Plus, research finds that some supplements contain many more milligrams than listed on the label (check with your pharmacist).

The best time to take a melatonin supplement is 30 to 60 minutes before bedtime. And because your body stores melatonin, the rule of thumb is to take supplements only when you need them.

Come morning, research finds that eating tryptophan-rich foods such as eggs and whole grains for breakfast and getting some daytime exposure to bright light promotes a healthy nighttime release of melatonin.

Sweet dreams.

Medical Warning: Consult with your doctor before taking melatonin supplements if you're pregnant, nursing, or taking antidepressants such as Prozac or Nardil.

Tip 40

Your Tongue is a Window Into Your Health

Many tongue disorders are linked to dehydration, nutrient deficiencies, prescription drugs, gut disorders, food allergies, inflammation, colds, or diseases.

During a checkup, doctors ask you to stick out your tongue to look for signs of illness. It lets them know by its color, moisture, coating, and papillae, which are tiny bumps of projecting tissues that contain your taste buds.

Therefore, changes in color, moisture, coating, or papillae can signal a short or a long-term health issue, making your tongue a window into your current health.

A healthy tongue should be evenly pink, moist, and slightly rough. One way to help diagnose some tongue disorders is to determine if your diet could have turned your tongue from a healthy pink to a potentially unhealthy grey (pale), white, yellow, or purple.

Tongue disorders such as grey tongue (a potential digestive issue, iron or B vitamin deficiency), white tongue (a potential dehydration, bacterial [yeast] infection, or B vitamin deficiency), yellow tongue (a potential excessive mucus, bacteria, or dead cells), and purple tongue (a potential poor circulation, iron, or red blood cell deficiency) can be helped, for example, by consuming iron-rich protein, fruits, vegetables, a vitamin B complex, drinking some organic apple cider vinegar and spring water, and daily exercise.

Furthermore, according to traditional Chinese medicine, the tongue is also known as a window into the health of your organs. Whereas the tip of your tongue is considered connected to your heart muscle; the tongue area above that to your lungs; the tongue center to your stomach and spleen; the tongue area above that to your small and large intestines; the tongue rear area to your kidneys, bladder, and glands; and the right and left sides of your tongue to your liver and gall bladder. So, accordingly, abnormal changes in these tongue areas can signal a potential health problem. For a tongue chart, search online for Traditional Chinese Medicine Tongue Diagnosis.

Studying your tongue to improve your health is an ongoing event. When yours quickly changes back to its evenly pink, moist, and slightly rough, it usually shows that your diet is working well. Though if you have any chronic tongue disorders, let your doctor know.

Tip 41

Beating Gout

Gout, the most common form of inflammatory arthritis, was once called the "Disease of Kings" for their overindulgence in rich foods and booze. It was first identified by the Egyptians in 2640 BCE and later recognized by Hippocrates in the fifth century who called it "the unwalkable disease." And depending on your lifestyle, you may be a risk now.

The first symptom of gout usually begins with swelling around a joint such as a big toe, ankle, or wrist. It then leads to redness, extreme tenderness, and pain to the point it's unbearable to touch—even with a feather—it can bring you to your knees! A friend once compared his gout pain to slamming a hammer on your big toe, twice.

And if left unchecked, it can lead to long-term consequences such as joint and tissue damage, kidney disorders, diabetes, heart failure, and even dementia.

Uric Acid and the Gout Connection

Gout is caused by hyperuricemia, an overabundance of uric acid, which causes needle-shaped salts called monosodium urate (MSU) crystals to form. Then, over time, these crystals build up and crystallize in or around a joint and let you know (loud and clear) with chronic inflammation—the extreme tenderness and pain known as a gout attack.

Most people, however, are unaware that gout might be around the corner for them because it can take months for enough MSU crystals to accumulate in a joint. But overnight, it can hit them like a hammer! In a lot of cases, gout first attacks the big toe (in the middle of the night). Although it's not uncommon for it to first attack the joints of the ankles, knees, elbows, wrists, or fingers.

Balancing Gout's Uric Acid Imbalance

Uric acid is a waste product of breaking down purine-containing foods such as red meat, liver, bacon, ham, chicken, turkey, sardines, anchovies, herring, crab, scallops, lobster, beer, and anything that contains high fructose corn syrup. It's then filtered through your kidneys and ends up in your urine; hence, the name uric acid.

Therefore, an important function of your kidneys is to maintain healthy uric acid levels. Uric acid is also a potent antioxidant and is considered to have neuroprotective properties; for instance, low levels are found in patients with multiple sclerosis, Parkinson's disease, and Alzheimer's disease. Though high levels are unhealthy.

So to balance a uric acid imbalance, reduce or eliminate the foods or drinks that give you gout or its symptoms.

Gout Prevention and Relief Tips

Here are some of the best tips to prevent and relieve gout:

- Drink a glass of lemon and spring water a few times a day. Its citric acid and vitamin C lowers uric acid levels.

- Take a 50 mg vitamin B complex. It metabolizes uric acid.

- Consume cucumbers, a diuretic that naturally eliminates uric acid.

- Drink 100% organic pure black cherry juice, which is the quickest and most effective remedy to prevent and relieve gout. Recommended by some doctors, black cherries contain a concentrated source of antioxidants and anti-inflammatory properties that reduce uric acid levels and quickly relieve gout's pain and swelling. I've seen it work numerous times. For quick relief, drink six ounces three times a day. Then to help prevent gout, continue to drink it daily. When purchasing, make sure the label states it contains 100% organic "pure" black cherry juice.

- Exercise daily. It reduces uric acid levels. Either walk fast, jog, swim, or engage in any physical activity that will get your heart pumping for at least 20 minutes a day.

Watching your diet and daily exercise is your ticket to living gout-free.

Tip 42

A Daily Parasite Protection Plan

Even the mention of a parasite sends chills up one's spine. Although many people don't think twice about them. They think that's something you only contract from visiting Third World countries. But the Centers for Disease Control and Prevention finds that millions of Americans host a parasite. And billions worldwide!

Parasites, as the name applies, cannot live on their own; they need a host like you to survive. Your options are to either ignore them or to take daily measures to prevent them from taking hold in the first place, which will improve your health in many ways. It's a vital part of achieving a disease-free life.

There are two main parasites: "protozoa" or single-celled parasites, including giardia, cryptosporidium, and Toxoplasma gondii that cannot be seen without a microscope. And "helminths" or multicellular parasites, including pinworms, tapeworms, and flatworms that can be seen with the naked eye.

Links Between Parasites and Diseases

Research links parasites, for instance, to Crohn's disease (Toxoplasma gondii parasite), colitis (whipworm parasite), celiac disease (hookworm parasite), epilepsy (tapeworm parasite), and cancers of the bladder, liver, and colon (flatworm parasite).

Amyotrophic lateral sclerosis (ALS), a.k.a. Lou Gehrig's disease, is also linked to the Toxoplasma gondii parasite that's mainly found in cat feces. According to researchers from the University of Virginia School of Medicine, over 2 billion people worldwide have the Toxoplasma gondii parasite, which is also linked to retardation. (Therefore, keep your cat indoors and daily clean the litter box.)

How People Contract Parasites

Most people contract parasites by consuming contaminated water, produce, or raw or undercooked beef, chicken, or fish. A sushi chef from Japan (the birthplace of sushi) once advised me never to eat raw sushi in a restaurant with a strong fishy smell because it's a telltale sign the fish is spoiled, making it a potential breeding ground for parasites.

Salad bars can be another breeding ground for parasites, bacteria, and germs. Some grow and flourish at temperatures between 40 to 140 degrees, known as the "Food Danger Zone." Thereby, salad bars are required to maintain the temperature of their cold foods below 40 degrees and their hot foods above 140 degrees. Either way, your body will usually let you know when you have eaten spoiled food (parasites). The first symptom is an upset stomach. Next is diarrhea.

And beware of pre-washed packages of vegetables. They can still carry parasites. So rinse them well.

Parasites are also found in or on the ground. Walking barefoot could expose you to one.

Again, you can contract parasites from animals. This usually happens when you accidentally touch their feces and then touch your mouth, nose, or eyes. For instance, if a dog rubs his butt on the carpet and you touch that area and then touch your mouth, you can become infected.

You can even contract a parasite by shaking someone's hand or touching a doorknob and then touching your mouth, nose, or eyes—so regularly wash hands.

Unprotected sex is another transmitter of parasites. And millions, of course, contract parasites from mosquitos, a carrier of the deadly malaria parasite and others.

Parasite Symptoms

Symptoms of hosting a parasite include anxiety, brain fog, poor memory, depression, chronic fatigue, malnutrition, grinding teeth, unexplained weight loss, indigestion, stomach cramps, food poisoning, ulcers, itchy anus, bloody or foul-smelling stools, diarrhea, and a loss of appetite.

The options to find out if you have a parasite include a stool test or a gut bacteria (microbiota) test. Ask your doctor for advise.

Naturally Preventing Parasites

Since we're all at risk of catching parasites, here's a natural parasite protection plan:

- Daily drink a tablespoon of organic apple cider vinegar in a glass of spring water. Its acetic acid, malic acid, and other properties help eliminate parasites. It also kills external parasites such as ringworm and athlete's foot by applying it to the infected area.

- Consume raw garlic. It contains antiparasitic properties that kill a variety of parasites including Toxoplasma gondii. Also consume raw onions, a cousin of garlic that contains similar parasite-preventing properties.

- Add some fresh oregano to your meal. It contains antiparasitic properties that help eliminate intestinal parasites.

- Add some turmeric to your meal. It contains antiparasitic properties that help eliminate intestinal worms.

- Drink clove tea or take a clove supplement. Cloves contain antiparasitic properties that remove intestinal parasites.

- Drink organic cranberry juice. Cranberries help prevent urinary tract infections by preventing the E. coli bug from adhering to the walls of your urinary tract. They also remove intestinal parasites.

- Eat a carrot or a sweet potato. They contain high levels of vitamin A that boost your immune defense system to protect against parasites.

- Take the supplement grapefruit seed extract, a natural antibiotic used to eliminate a wide range of parasites. Some doctors recommend it for severe parasitic infections. Although if taking prescription drugs, first consult with your doctor because consuming grapefruit with some pharmaceutical drugs strengthens the drug's potency.

- Take black walnut extract. It's one of the best supplements to kill intestinal worms, including tapeworms that can grow up to 80 feet long! Buy in tincture bottles and take as directed.

- Consume foods high in vitamin C. It helps inhibit the protozoa plasmodium parasite that causes malaria. Good food sources include lemons, oranges, mangos, broccoli, bell peppers, and parsley.

- Take a 15 mg zinc supplement. Zinc contains antiparasitic properties that kill intestinal parasites. Good food sources include seafood, lean meat, eggs, beans, peas, nuts, and seeds.

In short, here's a daily parasite protection plan: drink a tablespoon of organic apple cider vinegar in spring water, eat a carrot, sprinkle some raw garlic and oregano on your food, take a zinc supplement, and drink a glass of lemon and spring water.

Tip 43

Controlling Stress

Uncontrolled stress leads to memory loss and a smaller brain, according to the study, Circulating Cortisol and Cognitive and Structural Brain Measures. Researchers found a "Higher serum cortisol [the primary stress hormone] was associated with lower brain volumes and impaired memory in asymptomatic younger to middle-aged adults." Other research finds that stress shrinks your brain's hippocampus, where new memories are formed and transferred to long-term memory banks (the neocortex). It can also kill brain cells (neurons). So there's no doubt that your thoughts induce a biological impact on your overall health.

Research also finds that stress caused by "repetitive negative thinking" such as stressing out about the future or worrying about the past is linked to cognitive decline and higher amounts of neurofibrillary tangles and amyloid plaques, the two hallmarks of Alzheimer's disease.

Nevertheless, a high percentage of the population spends more time thinking this way than they do thinking about how to solve their real problems, which is perhaps the best remedy to reduce and control their stress levels. According to Earl Nightingale, who was known as the Dean of Personal Development and one of fifteen surviving marines on the USS Arizona on December 7, 1941, "No one is without problems [stress]; problems are a part of living. But let me show you how much time we waste in worrying about the wrong problems. Here's a reliable estimate of the things people worry about: things that never happen, 40 percent; things over and past that can't be changed by all the worry in the world, 30 percent; needless worries about our health, 12 percent; petty miscellaneous worries, 10 percent; real, legitimate worries, 8 percent. In short, 92 percent of the average person's worries take up valuable time, cause painful stress—even mental anguish—and are absolutely unnecessary."

Living with unhealthy levels of stress or worry is a mental drain or workout; it's like running a mental marathon over and over in your head. A well-regarded solution to overcoming and controlling stress is to have a positive mental outlook on life by thinking or dwelling less on negative thoughts and more on positive thoughts.

As the old proverb says, "You reap what you sow." So if you mainly reap negative thoughts, you will certainly sow or plant stress. But if you mainly reap positive thoughts, you will undoubtedly control stress. It can be as easy as that if you make it a habit, which takes around 21 days to form a new one. So don't give up.

How to Daily Change Your Thoughts to Control Your Stress Levels

Since you are what you think about, compile two lists to find out where you spend most of your thinking time. One list of all the negative thoughts (worries or problems) that come to mind. And one list of all the positive thoughts or goals. Go hour by hour.

Then the next time a negative thought pops into your mind (as it always will; it's human nature) replace it with a positive thought or goal from your positive list and act on it. The plan is to spend less time dwelling on negative thoughts and more time thinking and acting on positive thoughts, with the goal of living a more positive, productive, and stress-free life than a negative, unproductive, and stressed-out (worried) one. In other words, change your thoughts to change your life for the better.

To help you stay motivated, remember that prolonged stress or worry significantly increases your risk of premature aging and dementia. Research also finds that stress ages your immune system by reducing its T cells that guard against infections and diseases.

On the other hand, research finds that a positive or optimistic person who has learned how to control their stress levels looks and feels younger, has a healthier immune system, heart, and brain, and a lower risk of all-cause mortality.

Tip 44

Preventing and Reversing Gray Hairs

Research shows it's possible to prevent and reverse gray hairs with less stress and proper nutrition (at least some hairs).

First, your hair doesn't turn gray; it grows gray. As part of your body's natural renewal cycle, old hairs fall out and are replaced by the growth of new hairs, which is a key to keeping your natural hair color.

The Pigment Melanin Maintains Your Natural Hair Color

Your hair color is determined by a pigment called melanin produced in the melanocyte cells that surround the base of your hair follicles. Melanocyte cells inject melanin into keratin, the fibrous protein that forms hair, resulting in your hair color.

So having healthy melanocyte cells are a benchmark for holding on to your natural hair color. To protect them from deteriorating, the goal is to get into a daily habit of nourishing them. More on this to come.

Common Causes of Gray Hairs

It's not just old age or genes that can cause gray hairs. According to a Johns Hopkins University School of Medicine study, a diet of foods high in cholesterol and saturated fats causes skin inflammation, hair loss, and hair discoloration by affecting the proper function of melanocyte cells.

Consuming unhealthy fatty foods can also cause oxidative stress, a leading cause of gray hairs. Studies find that people with premature gray hair have a free radical and antioxidant imbalance.

Mental stress is another factor for it depletes melanocyte stem (master) cells, according to scientists from Harvard University and Harvard Stem Cell Institute.

Immune system and thyroid disorders are also linked to gray hairs.

And nutritional deficiencies can cause gray hairs. For instance, drinking too much coffee or any other high caffeine (diuretic) drink can lower iron, zinc, and B vitamin levels, which are required for maintaining normal hair color. Plus, alcohol can also lower B vitamins and other melanin nutrients.

A Gray Hair Prevention Diet

Here's an overview of the best foods and supplements that strengthen your hair and help prevent it from growing gray:

- Hair is protein. To increase levels of the protein keratin required for healthy hair structure, research recommends consuming wild salmon, trout, chicken, lean red meat, eggs, sweet potatoes, and Brewer's yeast.

- Vitamin A is needed for keratin synthesis. It also helps prevent dry skin and scalp. Good sources include apricots, cantaloupes, carrots, sweet potatoes, broccoli, kale, and spinach.

- The vitamin B7 biotin is also needed for keratin synthesis. Good sources include eggs, beef liver, wild salmon, sunflower seeds, almonds, sweet potatoes, and Brewer's yeast.

- Your thyroid gland plays a vital role in the growth and maintenance of your hair follicles. And since it requires the mineral iodine to function properly, low levels of iodine can cause gray hair and hair loss. Good sources of iodine include seaweed, kelp, cod, mussels, oysters, eggs, and black walnut hull extract. Or take a 150 mcg kelp supplement, the RDA.

- The amino acid tyrosine is required for producing melanin, the pigment that maintains your hair color. Good sources include fish, red meat, avocados, bananas, spinach, almonds, whole wheat bread, and Brewer's yeast.

- The mineral copper aids in the conversion of tyrosine to melanin. Good sources include shellfish, liver, avocados, mushrooms, chickpeas, cashews, sunflower seeds, and dark chocolate. Many multivitamins and some zinc supplements contain a safe ratio of 2 mg copper (RDA is 900 mcg) to 15 mg zinc (RDA is 11 mg for men; 8 mg for women).

- Zinc helps prevent gray hairs by aiding in producing

healthy new hairs (protein). Good sources include oysters, mussels, lean red meat, nuts, and seeds. To ensure you're getting your daily dosage, take a 15 mg zinc supplement.

- Omega-3 fatty acids are the healthy fats that help build and maintain the integrity of your melanocyte cells' membranes. They also aid with the production of keratin protein. Good sources include salmon, cod, sardines, shrimp, spinach, avocados, olive oil, flaxseeds, and walnuts. (See Tip 49 - Omega Fatty Acids Build and Maintain a Healthy Brain.)

- Iron, folate (vitamin B9), or vitamin B12 deficiency is also linked to gray hairs since they are vital for making healthy red blood cells that deliver oxygen to your hair follicles. Good sources of iron include dark green lettuce, spinach, asparagus, peas, unsulphured blackstrap molasses, lean red meat, liver, poultry, and clams. Good sources of folate include romaine lettuce, spinach, asparagus, broccoli, black-eyed peas, whole grains, peanuts, beef liver, and seafood. And good sources of vitamin B12 include red meat, clams, oysters, salmon, trout, tuna, poultry, egg yolks, and kidney beans. Or take a B12 sublingual supplement.

- The B vitamin para-aminobenzoic acid (PABA) has shown remarkable abilities to help restore hair to its original color by helping pigment metabolism. PABA is found in many vitamin B complex supplements. Good sources include Brewer's yeast, whole grains, mushrooms, and unsulphured blackstrap molasses.

- Unsulphured blackstrap molasses is a great gray hair remedy for it's a good source of PABA and iron. Add one to two tablespoons to a 1/2 cup of slightly heated spring water (to dissolve it) and stir well.

- The antioxidant catalase is considered the most important antioxidant to prevent gray hairs for it breaks down hydrogen peroxide, the reactive oxygen species (ROS free radicals) known to inhibit the production of melanin. Food sources include avocados, broccoli, kale, cabbage, sweet potatoes, onions, garlic, and Brewer's yeast.

- The antioxidant luteolin has been shown to reduce hair graying in mice. Good sources include celery, green peppers, hot peppers, broccoli, parsley, artichokes, apple skins, lemons, sage, thyme, and oregano.

- Brewer's yeast is perhaps the best all around gray hair remedy for it's a good source of the main hair color protecting nutrients: protein (keratin), biotin, tyrosine, copper, zinc, iron, folate, PABA, and catalase. Add a few tablespoons to a smoothie, juice, or cereal. (See Tip 47 - Brewer's Yeast: A Complete Meal.)

By applying these tips, at the least, your hair will be a lot healthier.

Tip 45

Resistance (Isometric) Exercises: A 20 Minute Workout and Detox Routine

Resistance exercises, also known as isometric (equal measurement) exercises, are a key to achieving overall strength and definition. You perform them by either holding or pushing a muscle into a state of resistance against another muscle or an unmovable object. And while doing so, you have also forced blood and fluid to circulate, which helps flush out toxins.

An advantage over most other workout routines is that you can do resistance exercises almost anywhere: at home, at the office, or at the local bar. And a complete routine only requires around 20 minutes of your time, three days a week, to increase and sustain muscle strength and definition.

Building Core Strength and Definition

Since gymnasts, wrestlers, and martial artists' training revolves around a state of resistance, they are prime examples of the inner-core strength and definition achievable through resistance muscle training.

Many professional bodybuilders also train with resistance exercises to further increase their overall strength and to define or cut their muscles. And during bodybuilding competitions, many perform flex-posing resistance exercises to maximize their pump and definition.

The good news is that it's never too late to start. According to the review, The Importance of Resistance Exercise Training to Combat Neuromuscular Aging, researchers found "age-related decrements in muscle health can benefit substantially from resistance exercise training, a potent stimulus for whole muscle and myofiber hypertrophy [breaking down fibers to rebuild stronger/bigger muscles], neuromuscular [nerve and muscle] performance gains, and improved functional mobility."

Resistance exercises are also highly recommended for injury rehabilitation. For instance, they help relieve lower back pain, improve muscle flexibility, and increase bone density. Other research found that isometric quadricep exercises can reduce osteoarthritis knee pain and improve muscle strength.

For best results, the goal is to use around 80% of your strength to hold a muscle or muscle group in a resistance position for 10 seconds, which is the right amount of time needed to break down muscle fibers. And performed correctly, it's always like completing that final important rep, for instance, on a bench press or a curl routine, also known as training to the point of momentary muscular failure, which achieves the greatest gains.

Resistance exercises also increase the break down of your muscle fibers at the angle they are performed, so train at different angles to break down a muscle group such as your chest muscles (more on this to come).

How Often Should I Workout?

After your muscle fibers break down, they need time to rebuild a stronger muscle. On average, it takes one to two days if you are under age 50 and two to three days if you are over 50 for your body to recover from a good workout. But if you don't rest enough, your results will be diminished because your muscle fibers cannot completely rebuild if they're still in a state of breaking down. As bodybuilders keenly understand, ample rest is a key to getting stronger and bigger.

Resistance Exercise Example

To help get you started, here's a resistance exercise example that strengthens and defines your chest muscles and cleavage: extend your arms straight out in front of your chest with your hands in the prayer position. Then push your hands together while focusing on tensing your chest muscles. Hold in that position (back straight) using 80% of your strength for 10 seconds—you should feel the tension in your chest muscles. And performed at different angles: arms extended in front of your body, above your head, and then straight down, breaks down your whole chest muscle fibers.

It's also important to keep breathing, especially if you have high blood pressure. Studies find that resistance exercise training helps control blood pressure, but anytime you perform any resistance exercise there is a tendency to hold your breath, which raises blood pressure. So if you have high blood pressure, take it easy. Nevertheless, resistance exercises will eventually build a stronger circulatory system that helps maintain healthy blood pressure.

Weekly Workout Example

Here's an example of a weekly workout routine that exercises practically all of your muscles. For best results, complete two or three sets of each exercise using at least 80% of your strength. Then rest for 30 seconds between sets. But first, warm up by stretching for at least 5 minutes.

Monday: Chest/Biceps/Stomach

1st Chest Exercise: Complete 10 floor push-ups. Then do a half push-up (elbows even to your shoulders) and hold in that position for 10 seconds. Rest and repeat.

2nd Chest Exercise: As described in the workout example, extend your arms straight out in front of your chest with your hands in the prayer position. Then push your hands together and tense your chest muscles for 10 seconds. Rest and repeat at different angles, from above your head to below it.

1st Biceps Exercise: Flex (tense) your biceps muscles for 10 seconds. Rest and repeat.

2nd Biceps Exercise: Sit at a desk and place both hands (palms up) underneath the desktop. Then with your back straight, try to lift the desk up with your bicep muscles. Think of it as doing a half dumbbell curl. But don't lift the desk. Instead, the goal is to put the right amount of resistance load on your biceps muscles without lifting it. Breathe and hold for 10 seconds. Rest and repeat. Good posture is essential to prevent back strain.

1st Stomach Exercise: Sit at a desk and straighten your arms and place the palms of your hands on top of the desk. Then with your back straight, push down on your palms while tensing your stomach muscles. Hold for 10 seconds. Rest and repeat.

2nd Stomach Exercise: Lie on the floor in the sit-up position: flat on your back with your knees up and hands together behind the back of your head. Then do a half sit-up, a.k.a. a sit-up crunch. Hold in that position (stomach tensed) for 10 seconds. Rest and repeat.

Wednesday: Legs/Shoulders

1st Thighs Exercise: Complete 10 leg squats. Then squat halfway down and hold for 10 seconds. Rest and repeat.

2nd Thighs Exercise: Sit in a chair and bend forward enough to place your arms' elbows next to the outside of your knee caps. Then try to push your knees outward while using the resistance of your arms to prevent this movement. Concentrate on using your legs to do the work instead of your arms; your arms act as a barrier against your legs moving. Hold for 10 seconds. Rest and repeat. Next, place your elbows inside of your knee caps. Then try to push the knees together while using the resistance of your arms to prevent this movement. Rest and repeat. Again, don't forget to breathe.

Hamstrings Exercise: Find a coffee table, bed, or another low laying object that allows you to stand with your back facing it and the back of your foot underneath it. Then try to lift, for example, a coffee table up with your hamstring muscle (not your foot) and hold for 10 seconds. Rest and repeat. Then repeat with your other hamstring muscle.

Calfs Exercise: Rise up on your toes and tense your calf muscles. Then hold for 10 seconds. Rest and repeat.

1st Shoulders Exercise: Stand underneath a door frame and put your hands on the top of the frame (some will need a stool). Then using your shoulder muscles, push straight up and hold for 10 seconds. Think of it as pressing a barbell over your head and holding it. Rest and repeat.

2nd Shoulders Exercise: While standing underneath a door frame, put your arms straight down and place the backside of your hands against the sides of the door frame. Then using your deltoid (top) shoulder muscles, try to raise your arms up. Hold for 10 seconds. Rest and repeat.

3rd Shoulders Exercise: Roll up a towel and grab it with both hands at around shoulder length. Then lift the towel over your head and try to pull it apart for 10 seconds. Next, put the towel in front of your chest and try to pull it apart. Then put the towel behind your back and try to pull it apart. Rest and repeat each exercise.

Friday: Latissimus Dorsi (Lats)/Triceps/Hands

1st Lats Exercise: Find a dresser drawer that's about chest high and four feet wide. Next, place the palms of your hands on the outside of the dresser as if you're trying to hug it. Then using your back lat muscles, push in from each side. Hold for 10 seconds. Rest and repeat.

2nd Lats Exercise: Stand under a door frame with your hands clenched into fists and put the backside of them against the sides of the door frame. Then using your lat muscles, push in on each side. Hold for 10 seconds. Rest and repeat.

3rd Lats Exercise: Sit at a desk and straighten your arms and place the palms of your hands on top of the desk. Then using the muscles of your lats (instead of your stomach muscles), push down for 10 seconds. To target the long vertical muscles of your lats, vary the position of the hands on the desk from close together to far apart. Rest and repeat each exercise position.

Triceps Exercise: Sit at a desk and make two fists and place them on the top of the desk. Then using your tricep muscle, push down and hold for 10 seconds. Rest and repeat.

Hands/Forearms Exercise: Grab two tennis balls. Then squeeze hard for 10 seconds. Rest and repeat.

Hands/Fingers Exercise: Grab your hands together with your fingers (elbows out or horizontal) and then try to pull them apart for 10 seconds. Rest and repeat. Then reverse hand positions and repeat. This is also a great exercise for strengthening the shoulder muscles. But to mainly increase hand and finger strength, concentrate on pulling with just your fingers. That applies to all resistance exercises: for maximum results, concentrate on using just that muscle or muscle group.

Since you now have a general idea of how to perform resistance exercises, try making up your own. For instance, to exercise your neck muscles, place a fist under your chin and push down with your neck muscles while pushing up equally with your fist. Plus, flexing any muscle will achieve the same results. There are also many resistance (isometric) exercise examples online.

Resistance exercises also release endorphins. So after a workout, you'll look stronger (pumped) and feel better too.

Tip 46

Why We Need Sunshine (Vitamin D)

The sun gives us internal health and vitality; we really can't live without it. The only thing you should never do is look directly at it—for it can blind you! Its health benefits date to the father of modern medicine, Hippocrates, who prescribed sunbaths to treat a variety of aliments, including depression.

A lack of sunshine (vitamin D) is also linked to impaired thinking, memory loss, fatigue, weak bones and muscles, slow wound healing, and sleeping problems.

The Sunshine and Vitamin D Link

Vitamin D is nicknamed the "Sunshine Vitamin" because it is naturally produced in your skin by exposure to the sun's ultraviolet B (UVB) rays. It's then converted by your liver into 25-hydroxyvitamin D, which your body also stores. Next, your kidneys convert it into 1,25 dihydroxyvitamin D or calcitriol, the active hormonal form of vitamin D. (Although a 25-hydroxyvitamin D test is the most accurate way to measure your current vitamin D levels because its circulating levels are greater than 1,25 dihydroxyvitamin D levels.)

Vitamin D is most known for building strong bones by maintaining proper calcium and phosphorus levels. But it also improves immune, cardiovascular, liver, kidney, gut, lung, and endocrine (hormone) functions. It's also a potent antioxidant that protects against hypertension, infectious diseases, diabetes, arthritis, dementia, and some forms of cancer. A US Navy study on melanoma risk, for example, found that naval personnel showed a much higher risk of melanoma (the deadliest form of skin cancer) among those with indoor jobs than those working outside in the sunlight.

Around a billion people worldwide have a vitamin D deficiency due to a lack of sunlight. And an "increasing numbers of Americans suffer from vitamin D deficiencies and serious health problems caused by insufficient sun exposure…The message of sun avoidance must be changed to acceptance of non-burning sun exposure sufficient to achieve serum 25(OH)D [25-hydroxyvitamin D] concentration of 30 ng/mL [approximately 1000 IU] or higher in the sunny season," according to the review, The Risks and Benefits of Sun Exposure 2016.

Though many are in jeopardy of a vitamin D deficiency just by where they live. Studies find that those living in the northern regions of the earth (above the 37th parallel north that runs in the US from Northern California to Virginia) are more prone to a vitamin D deficiency in the fall and winter months or between October to March. During this time, the sun is not high enough in the northern sky for its UVB rays to produce adequate amounts of vitamin D. Instead, the sun is in the southern sky.

So northerners need to increase their vitamin D intake from October to March or when the sun's rays are least intense.

RDA for Vitamin D

The RDA for vitamin D is 800 IU (International Units) for adults. Although the Endocrine Society and other experts recommend 1500 IU to 2000 IU a day for adults and 1000 IU a day for children, which may become the future RDA.

Here is a breakdown of vitamin D calculated on sun exposure, according to the review, Benefits of Sunlight: A Bright Spot for Human Health. "For most white people, a half-hour in the summer sun in a bathing suit can initiate the release of 50,000 IU (1.25 mg) vitamin D into the circulation within 24 hours of exposure; this same amount of exposure yields 20,000–30,000 IU in tanned individuals and 8,000–10,000 IU in dark-skinned people."

Therefore, most only need sun exposure for 10 to 15 minutes a few times a week in a t-shirt to maintain healthy levels. Then when their body needs more, their vitamin D storage banks (fat tissues) will release more.

Regarding indoor sunlight, the "UVB radiation does not penetrate glass, so exposure to sunshine indoors through a window does not produce vitamin D," according to the National Institutes of Health (NIH).

If you don't receive your weekly required sunshine, then take a vitamin D supplement or consume vitamin D-rich foods.

Vitamin D Foods

The best food sources of vitamin D include cod liver oil, wild salmon, herring, sardines, oysters, and eggs.

To help increase your vitamin D absorption, consume

magnesium-rich foods, according to the study, Magnesium Status and Supplementation Influence Vitamin D Status and Metabolism: Results From a Randomized Trial. "Our findings suggest that optimal magnesium status may be important for optimizing 25(OH)D [25-hydroxyvitamin D] status." The best food sources of magnesium include whole wheat bread, black beans, almonds, peanuts, cashews, pumpkin seeds, bananas, avocados, and spinach.

The Best Vitamin D Supplement

There are two main vitamin D supplements: vitamin D2 (ergocalciferol) that's made from invertebrates, fungus, and plants, although it has a lower absorption rate. The other is vitamin D3 (cholecalciferol) that's made from sheep's wool and instead has a higher absorption rate and therefore is considered the best source next to sun exposure, according to the study, Long-Term Vitamin D3 Supplementation is More Effective Than Vitamin D2 in Maintaining Serum 25-Hydroxyvitamin D Status Over the Winter Months. So look for a vitamin D3 supplement instead of vitamin D2.

Tanning Beds and Sun Lamps Alert

It's possible to get some vitamin D from lying on a tanning bed or with a sun lamp, but research finds their artificial UV radiation significantly increases your risk of melanoma skin cancer.

In 2009, the World Health Organization's International Agency for Research on Cancer added tanning beds and sun lamps to its highest cancer risk category: Carcinogenic to Humans. They found that they are as dangerous as arsenic and mustard gas.

Concerns with Sunscreen Lotions

Sunscreen lotions do what their name applies: they help block the sun's rays from properly penetrating your skin, but they also help block vitamin D from properly synthesizing. As a result, millions of people have a vitamin D deficiency due to sunscreen use, according to the study, Vitamin D Deficiency, Its Role in Health and Disease, and Current Supplementation Recommendations. Researchers found that using a SPF (Sun Protection Factor) 15 or higher reduces vitamin D3 production by 99 percent! Therefore, the FDA should require sunscreen lotions to contain a "health warning label" stating that they cause a vitamin D deficiency.

Plus, some of the approved FDA ingredients found in many sunscreen lotions contain chemicals linked to hormonal problems, such as oxybenzone, avobenzone, and homosalate. So if you plan on tanning, purchase an all-natural sunscreen lotion. And to help protect you from sunshine's free radicals (the double-edged sword), take a grape seed extract supplement and drink some iced green tea.

There's nothing like a sunny day to lift one's spirits. It's also an effective remedy for shaking off a hangover. Besides helping to sweat out alcohol, the sun's rays help you feel better by upping your endorphin and serotonin levels.

Tip 47

Brewer's Yeast: A Complete Meal

This tip is about a popular Brewer's yeast strain called Saccharomyces cerevisiae that's used to make a great beer and a great nutritional yeast supplement. And like beer, it makes you feel good too.

It's also a complete meal. Just two tablespoons of a high-quality brand (e.g., Saccharomyces cerevisiae grown or fermented on sugar beet molasses) contain a significant source of protein, B vitamins, antioxidants, dietary fiber, and the minerals potassium, copper, zinc, selenium, and chromium, the key mineral that regulates glucose (sugar) levels to help prevent hyperglycemia (high blood sugar) and hypoglycemia (low blood sugar).

Protein

Brewer's yeast is one of the best sources of protein (amino acids). Just two tablespoons of a high-quality supplement contain approximately 14 grams or 25% of the RDA for an average size adult. And it not only contains the nine essential amino acids required to be a complete source of protein but also the eleven nonessential amino acids; you need a boost from them sometimes too.

Its amino acids phenylalanine, tyrosine, and tryptophan also boost your dopamine and serotonin levels.

B Vitamins

Brewer's yeast is also one of the best sources of the seven essential B vitamins: B1 thiamin, B2 riboflavin, B3 niacin, B5 pantothenic acid, B6 pyridoxine hydrochloride, B7 biotin, and B9 folic. It's only lacking vitamin B12 cobalamin to qualify as a vitamin B complex or containing the eight essential B vitamins (although fortified nutritional yeast brands contain B12 cyanocobalamin, its synthetic form). It's also a good source of the three non-essential B vitamins: choline, inositol, and PABA.

B vitamins are needed for healthy digestion, energy production, brain function, and for helping to prevent and relieve a hangover. (See Tip 30 - Importance of Vitamin B Complex.)

Antioxidants

Brewer's yeast increases your defense antioxidants superoxide dismutase, catalase, and glutathione (the master antioxidant), which is synthesized from its amino acids cysteine, glutamic acid, and glycine. It also contains polyphenol antioxidants.

Plus, it's a good source of alpha lipoic acid (the universal antioxidant) that also helps regenerate glutathione and the antioxidants vitamin E, vitamin C, and coenzyme Q10 (CoQ10), which is also found in Brewer's yeast. CoQ10 also strengthens your heart muscle and protects against congestive heart failure.

Fiber

Brewer's yeast is also one of the best sources of fiber. Just two tablespoons of a high-quality yeast brand contain approximately six grams or 20% of the RDA, making it a constipation remedy. It also contains beta-glucan fiber, a heart-healthy soluble fiber (prebiotic) that research finds to boost your gut microbes' immune defenses against the common cold and flu and relieves the duration of their symptoms, making its fiber also a cold and flu prevention remedy.

Dosage

Brewer's yeast (Saccharomyces cerevisiae) brands grown on non-GMO sugar beet molasses (e.g., Bluebonnet, Lewis Labs) contain the highest levels of nutrients. Two large tablespoons a day is all you need for a meal. Add it to your protein shake, mix it with grape juice, or sprinkle it on your cereal; most brands now have a nutty taste.

Brewer's yeast is also inactive, so it won't cause a yeast overgrowth in your body. It can, however, interact with some medications such as monoamine oxidase inhibitors (anti-depression medications), Demerol (a narcotic pain medication), and some diabetes medications.

Start or end your day with a boost of Brewer's yeast, a healthy feel-good meal that also helps overcome a hangover.

Tip 48

Berries Are Brain Food

Studies find that berries such as blueberries, bilberries, blackberries, mulberries, raspberries, and strawberries contain a rich source of flavonoid antioxidants and anti-inflammatory properties that protect your brain cells or neurons from oxidative stress (a leading cause of dementia) while improving their cell signaling and connections.

Your brain contains around 100 billion neurons that make 100 trillion connections. They are your so-called excitable nerve cells that receive and transmit information throughout your brain and body by a process called electrochemical signaling. Whereas berries help enhance neuroplasticity, or your brain's ability to form new neuron connections. They also energize the birth of new neurons.

Scientists at the USDA Human Nutrition Research Center on Aging at Tufts University fed aging rats a blueberry, spinach, or strawberry dietary supplement and found "that nutritional intervention with fruits and vegetables may play an important role in reversing the deleterious effects of aging on neuronal function and behavior." So you can teach an old rat new tricks after all.

And the "daily consumption of wild blueberries is shown here to improve speed of [cognitive] processing, especially in those 75–80 years of age," according to the study, Six-Month

Intervention with Wild Blueberries Improved Speed of Processing in Mild Cognitive Decline: A Double-Blind, Placebo-Controlled, Randomized Clinical Trial, which included 86 adults between the ages of 65 and 80.

Furthermore, "this systematic review provides evidence for the beneficial effects of berry anthocyanins [antioxidants] on cognitive performance as memory was improved," according to the study, Effects of Berry Anthocyanins on Cognitive Performance, Vascular Function and Cardiometabolic Risk Markers: A Systematic Review of Randomized Placebo-Controlled Intervention Studies in Humans, which included 49 randomized placebo-controlled intervention studies.

Other studies find that the variety of antioxidants found in berries, such as anthocyanins and quercetin, reduces your risk of Parkinson's disease and Alzheimer's disease. They also help extend your life span by lowering your risks of cardiovascular diseases and cancer. And they help increase lung function and protect smokers against lung disorders.

Berries are also a good source of fiber, complex carbohydrates, and vitamin C.

Organic Berries

Non-organic or conventional berries usually rank high in pesticides, so whenever possible, buy organic berries.

A handful of berries a day keeps the neurologist away.

Tip 49

Omega Fatty Acids Build and Maintain a Healthy Brain

The omega fatty acids, the polyunsaturated fatty acids, are called the "essential fatty acids" because your brain (and body) requires them to function properly but can't make them.

They are essential, for instance, for building and maintaining a larger gray matter volume, the outermost layer of your brain that houses your estimated 100 billion brain cells or neurons. Among its many functions, your gray matter processes sensory information, controls movement, retains memories, and regulates emotions. They also help build a larger hippocampal (hippocampus) volume that plays a major role in learning and memory. And they improve intercellular signaling and blood flow to the brain needed for increasing brainpower.

The omega fatty acids are also essential for building healthy brain cell membranes (lipids), which are required to protect their cellular integrity; many neurological disorders have their roots in dysfunctional cell membranes, including Alzheimer's disease. And after consuming them, they are soon incorporated into your cell membranes (as with unhealthy fats); measurable changes in cellular membrane structure can occur within days of regular consumption.

So the key to an overall healthier brain structure and brain cells is to consume healthy omega fatty acids rather than unhealthy saturated fats and artificial trans fats (hydrogenated fats) that instead harm gray (and white) matter structure and brain cells by hardening membranes, increasing your risk of neurological disorders. In other words, since new cells are born daily, you want them built out of healthy omega fatty acids instead of unhealthy fats.

Other research finds that omega fatty acids help prevent depression, dementia, anxiety disorders, bipolarism, and attention deficit hyperactivity disorder (ADHD). Scientists have known for years that a child deficient in omega-3 fatty acids has a smaller gray matter volume and is more prone to learning and behavioral problems.

They also "exerted beneficial effects on white matter microstructural integrity…[and] better axonal transmission," according to the study, Long-Chain Omega-3 Fatty Acids Improve Brain Function and Structure in Older Adults.

The omega fatty acids also help build and maintain a healthy white matter, the other half of your brain that houses your intertwining wiring network of millions of axons (nerve fibers). An axon is a neuron's long threadlike fiber that's used to communicate with other neurons and gray matter by transmitting electrical and chemical neurotransmitter signals. Hence, healthy white matter is vital for fast mental processing and a higher intelligence. And "lower brain-wide white matter tract integrity exerts a substantial negative effect on general intelligence through reduced information-processing speed," according to the study, Brain White Matter Tract Integrity as a Neural Foundation for General Intelligence. So there's also a condition called white matter dementia.

Breaking Down the Omega Fatty Acids: The Omega-3 Fatty Acids

There are three omega-3 fatty acids that are most important or essential: alpha-linolenic acid (ALA), which is found in plant foods such as green leafy vegetables, broccoli, kale, spinach, avocados, whole grains, beans, walnuts, hazelnuts, pecans, pumpkin seeds, flaxseeds, hemp seeds, and olive oil. And eicosapentaenoic acid (EPA) and docosahexaenoic acid (DHA), which are found in marine and freshwater fish such as rainbow trout, bass, wild salmon, sardines, anchovies, halibut, herring, cod, tuna, oysters, clams, and shrimp. (EPA and DHA can also be derived from ALA, but the conversion rate is low.)

Alpha-linolenic acid and eicosapentaenoic acid are most known for building a healthy immune system and reducing inflammation. They also help relieve depression by stimulating and improving the functions of your neurotransmitters, including acetylcholine, dopamine, and serotonin. Whereas docosahexaenoic acid also reduces inflammation and improves neurotransmitter functions, but is most known for helping to build and maintain a healthy brain structure, central nervous system, and retinas, making DHA the vital omega fatty acid for the growth and development of a healthy child.

Consuming omega-3 fatty acids is also "robustly associated with lower mortality from major causes," according to the study, Association of Fish and Long-Chain Omega-3 Fatty Acids Intakes With Total and Cause-Specific Mortality: Prospective Analysis of 421,309 Individuals. So those with higher blood levels of omega-3 fatty acids also have better odds of living longer too.

A groundbreaking 2010 study from the University of California, San Francisco, found that coronary heart disease patients with high levels of omega-3 fatty acids increased their survival rate by slowing the shortening of their telomeres. Telomeres are the ends of chromosomes (DNA molecules) that have been compared to the plastic caps on the ends of shoelaces, which prevent them from fraying. But every time a cell divides (around every 24 hours), its telomeres shorten and the rate of which increases your risk of DNA aging. If you are curious, there's a telomere test that tries to determine your biological age by the current length of your telomeres.

The Omega-6 Fatty Acids (and the Omega-3 Fatty Acids Imbalance Problem)

The other essential fatty acids are the omega-6 fatty acids, which are derived from linolenic acid (LA), the parent of alpha-linolenic acid (ALA). So as with omega-3 fatty acids, research finds that omega-6 fatty acids also helps build a healthy brain and are heart healthy. A healthy intake of omega fatty acids is considered between a 1:1 to 4:1 ratio of omega-6 fatty acids to omega-3 fatty acids. Good sources of omega-6 fatty acids include eggs, oats, beans, almonds, peanut butter, walnuts, flaxseeds, hemp seeds, sunflower seeds, avocados, olive oil, and evening primrose oil.

But there's an omega fatty acid imbalance problem: too many people are consuming an estimated 15:1 ratio of omega-6 fatty acids to omega-3 fatty acids, which is easy to reach since omega-6 fatty acids are also found in red meat, fried foods, baked goods, crackers, margarine, soybean oil, corn oil, sunflower oil, and canola oil.

A higher intake of omega-6 fatty acids is harmful because it can create an abundance of arachidonic acid, a linolenic acid that's well-known to promote inflammation (for vital immune responses) but too much increases your risk of inflammatory arthritis, cardiovascular diseases, and neurological disorders. Plus, consuming too many omega-6 fatty acids reduces your omega-3 fatty acid levels.

So to reach a healthy omega fatty acids ratio or balance, the goal is to consume fewer foods high in omega-6 fatty acids, such as red meat, fried foods, and processed foods, and more foods high in omega-3 fatty acids, such as seafood, green leafy vegetables, and nuts.

Symptoms of an omega-3 fatty acids deficiency include depression, dry skin, gray hair, hair loss, and poor wound healing.

What About Fish Oil Pills or Bottled-Up Omega-3 Fatty Acids?

Another way to get your omega-3 fatty acids (EPA and DHA) is to take a fish oil supplement. Though the medical jury is still out on their effectiveness, studies seem to weigh in their favor. For instance, a 2020 large cohort study of 427,678 men and women found the habitual use of fish oil seems to lower the risk of all-cause cardiovascular mortality.

But to make fish oil, some companies cheat and use substandard fish that contains toxins linked to health disorders. The solution is to buy fish oil supplements that state on their label or close to it: "Free of detectable levels of mercury, cadmium, lead, PCBs (polychlorinated biphenyls), and other contaminants." (Many farmed-raised salmon are also high in cancer-linked PCBs via their diet of contaminated fishmeal.)

Besides fish oil, other oil sources of omega-3 fatty acids include krill oil, algal oil, and cod liver oil. It's also important to refrigerate oil supplements to help prevent them from turning rancid.

Recommended Allowance

Research recommends consuming approximately 1500 mg (EPA 500 mg/DHA 1000 mg) of omega-3 fatty acids per serving. This equals, for example, around three ounces of wild salmon. And because your body stores healthy fats, take it easy on the fish oil pills. Consuming fresh or frozen fish three or four times a week is ideal.

But avoid consuming fish high in mercury more than a few times a month since mercury poisoning causes neurological disorders. Fish high in mercury (higher amounts in larger fish) include swordfish, shark, marlin, king mackerel, tuna (albacore, Bigeye), tilefish, Chilean sea bass, and grouper. Fish low in mercury include anchovies, sardines, wild salmon, flounder, trout, cod, pollock, sole, and shrimp.

And remember it's also important to consume foods that maintain healthy levels of the essential alpha-linolenic acid (an omega-3 fatty acid) and linolenic acid (an omega-6 fatty acid), such as green leafy vegetables, broccoli, kale, avocados, whole grains, beans, almonds, walnuts, sunflower seeds, flaxseeds, and olive oil.

The omega fatty acids also help you recover quicker from a hangover by decreasing inflammation and increasing your ability to absorb and retain nutrients. They're also essential for energy production.

Tip 50

Brain Cells Regrow After All

Studies find that the human brain produces new brain cells (neurons) by a process called neurogenesis, the regeneration or regrowth of new neurons. This is great news for all who were raised on the old belief that we were born with all the brain cells we were ever going to have, unlike your other cells (mainly red blood cells) that are born daily.

For instance, "In adult humans, 700 new neurons are added per day [to the hippocampal, the two hippocampus seahorse-shaped memory centers]," according to the study, Dynamics of Hippocampal Neurogenesis in Adult Humans. Researchers "conclude that neurons are generated throughout adulthood and that the rates are comparable in middle aged humans and mice, suggesting that adult hippocampal neurogenesis may contribute to human brain function."

So for anyone who thinks they may be suffering from brain damage, there's still hope!

Neurogenesis: A Brief History of the Evidence

- 1962 to 1983: The paper, Brain Basics: The Life & Death of a Neuron by the US National Institute of Neurological Disorders and Stroke, found "Until recently, most neuroscientists thought we were born with all the neurons we were ever going to have…In 1962, scientist Joseph Altman challenged this belief when he saw evidence of neurogenesis in a region of the adult rat brain called the hippocampus. He later reported that newborn neurons migrated from their birthplace in the hippocampus to other parts of the brain. In 1979, scientist Michael Kaplan confirmed Altman's findings in the rat brain, and in 1983 he found neural precursor cells in the forebrain of an adult monkey."

- 1998: The study, Neurogenesis in the Adult Human Hippocampus, found "that cell genesis occurs in human brains and that the human brain retains the potential for self-renewal throughout life."

- 1999: The study, Neurogenesis in the Neocortex of Adult Primates, found "new neurons, which are continually added in adulthood, may play a role in the functions of association neocortex [the center for memory, sight, hearing, language, perception, and reasoning]."

- 2018: The study, Human Hippocampal Neurogenesis Persists Throughout Aging, researchers "assessed whole autopsy hippocampi from healthy human individuals ranging from 14 to 79 years of age. We found similar numbers of intermediate neural progenitors and thousands of immature neurons."

- 2019: The study, Adult Hippocampal Neurogenesis is Abundant in Neurologically Healthy Subjects and Drops Sharply in Patients With Alzheimer's Disease (AD), also "demonstrate the persistence of AHN [adult hippocampal neurogenesis] during both physiological and pathological aging in humans and provide evidence for impaired neurogenesis as a potentially relevant mechanism underlying memory deficits in AD that might be amenable to novel therapeutic strategies."

These studies and others have given new hope for treating brain diseases. In the future, for instance, scientists may be able to cure dementia by channeling neural stem cells to repair the damage.

What Harms Brain Cells the Most?

Besides exposure to chemicals, pesticides, and heavy metals (e.g., aluminum, cadmium, lead, and mercury), research finds that stress harms your brain cells the most. Stress also disrupts your brain cells' homeostasis. And chronic stress causes the loss of brain cell connections (synapses), reducing brain volume. It can also kill brain cells.

Foods for a Healthier Brain

Research finds that consuming inflammatory foods or foods that contain refined carbohydrates, sugars, salt, and saturated fats are linked to a smaller brain volume and a higher risk of brain disorders. Whereas consuming anti-inflammatory foods such as fruits, vegetables, whole grains, and fish are linked to a larger brain volume (including a larger gray matter volume, hippocampal volume, and white matter volume) and a lower risk of brain disorders.

For brain protection, the antioxidants found in fruits, vegetables, whole grains, nuts, seeds, herbs, and teas are able to cross your very selective blood-brain barrier (BBB) to protect it from free radicals and oxidative stress, the underlying cause of many neurological disorders.

To increase your brain's mood-enhancing neurotransmitters, consume seafood, turkey, berries, bananas, mangos, lemons, avocados, broccoli, kale, cauliflower, almonds, walnuts, sunflower seeds, pumpkin seeds, flaxseeds, dark chocolate, and hot peppers.

Exercise Improves Brainpower

Exercise is also a great way to strengthen your brainpower, according to the study, Exercise Training Increases the Size of Hippocampus and Improves Memory. Researchers found in "a randomized controlled trial with 120 older adults, that aerobic exercise training increases the size of the anterior hippocampus, leading to improvements in spatial memory. Exercise training increased hippocampal volume by 2%, effectively reversing age-related loss in volume by 1 to 2 y."

Plus, peak oxygen uptake helps increase gray matter tissue, according to the study, Cardiorespiratory Fitness [CRF] and Gray Matter [GM] Volume in the Temporal, Frontal, and Cerebellar Regions in the General Population. Researchers "suggest that CRF might contribute to improved brain health and might, therefore, decelerate pathology-specific GM decrease." Do any exercise that gets your heart pumping for at least 20 minutes a day, such as walking fast, jogging, biking, or swimming.

Exercise also boost your neurotransmitters.

Brain Exercises

Research finds that having a positive mental outlook on life and learning new skills increase and improve your brain cell connections and long-term memory. Therefore, stay positive and push your intellect, for instance, through memory tasks, crossword puzzles, chess, writing, studying, and reading. As the English writer and poet Joseph Addison (1672-1719) reminds us: "Reading is to the mind, what exercise is to the body."

References

Introduction

1. Lukasz Aleksandrowicz, Phillip Baker, Komal Bhatia, et al. Food systems and diets: Facing the challenges of the 21st century. Global Panel on Agriculture and Food Systems for Nutrition. 2016.
2. Ashkan Afshin, Patrick John Sur, Kairsten A Fay, et al. Health effects of dietary risks in 195 countries, 1990-2017: a systematic analysis for the Global Burden of Disease Study 2017. Lancet. 2019.
3. Paul M Johnson and Paul J Kenny. Dopamine D2 receptors in addiction-like reward dysfunction and compulsive eating in obese rats. Nature Neuroscience. 2010.
4. Chronic Diseases in America. CDC National Center for Chronic Disease and Health Promotion. 2022.
5. Nicola P. Bondonna, Frederik Dalgaard, Cecilie Kyrø, et al. Flavonoid intake is associated with lower mortality in the Danish Diet Cancer and Health Cohort. Nature Communications. 2019.
6. Youjin Kim, Tianxiao Huan, Roby Joehanes, et al. Higher diet quality relates to decelerated epigenetic aging. The American Journal of Clinical Nutrition. 2021.
7. Bo Xi, Sreenivas P. Veeranki, Min Zhao, Chuanwei Ma, et al. Relationship of Alcohol Consumption to All-Cause, Cardiovascular (CV), and Cancer-Related Mortality in U.S. Adults. Journal of the American College of Cardiology. 2017.

Tip 1 - Antioxidants: Winning the Anti-Aging Battle Against Free Radicals and Oxidative Stress

1. Bee Ling Tan, Mohd Esa Norhaizan, Winnie-Pui-Pui Liew, and Heshu Sulaiman Rahman. Antioxidant and Oxidative Stress: A Mutual Interplay in Age-Related Diseases. Frontiers in Pharmacology. 2018.
2. Lien Ai Pham-Huy, Hua He, and Chuong Pham-Huy. Free Radicals, Antioxidants in Disease and Health. International Journal of Biomedical Science. 2008.
3. T M Florence. The role of free radicals in disease. Australian and New Zealand Journal of Ophthalmology. 1995.
4. Alugoju Phaniendra, Dinesh Babu Jestadi, and Latha Periyasamy. Free Radicals: Properties, Sources, Targets, and Their Implication in Various Diseases. Indian Journal of Clinical Biochemistry. 2015.
5. V. Lobo, A. Patil, A. Phatak, and N. Chandra. Free radicals, antioxidants and functional foods: Impact on human health. Pharmacognosy. 2010.
6. Borut Poljšak and Raja Dahmane. Free Radicals and Extrinsic Skin Aging. Dermatology Research and Practice. 2012.
7. J P Silva, O P Coutinho. Free radicals in the regulation of damage and cell death - basic mechanisms and prevention. Drug Discoveries & Therapeutics. 2010.
8. Maura Lodovici and Elisabetta Bigagli. Oxidative Stress and Air Pollution Exposure. Journal of Toxicology. 2011.
9. Suzana Saric and Raja K. Sivamani. Polyphenols and Sunburn. International Journal of Molecular Sciences. 2016.
10. Parul Chauhan, H N Verma, Rashmi Sisodia, Kavindra Kumar Kesari. Microwave radiation (2.45 GHz)-induced oxidative stress: Whole-body exposure effect on histopathology of Wistar rats. Electromagnetic Biology and Medicine. 2016.
11. Elcin Ozgur, Göknur Güler, Nesrin Seyhan. Mobile phone radiation-induced free radical damage in the liver is inhibited by the antioxidants N-acetyl cysteine and epigallocatechin-gallate. International Journal of Radiation Biology. 2010.
12. Bevelacqua J. J., Mehdizadeh A. R., and Mortazavi S. M. J. A New Look at Three Potential Mechanisms Proposed for the Carcinogenesis of 5G Radiation. The Journal of Biomedical Physics and Engineering. 2020.
13. Stefania Schiavone, Vincent Jaquet, Luigia Trabace, and Karl-

Heinz Krause. Severe Life Stress and Oxidative Stress in the Brain: From Animal Models to Human Pathology. Antioxidants & Redox Signaling. 2013.

14. Fehmi Ozguner, Ahmet Koyu, Gokhan Cesur. Active smoking causes oxidative stress and decreases blood melatonin levels. Toxicology and Industrial Health. 2005.

15. Damian G. Deavall, Elizabeth A. Martin, Judith M. Horner, and Ruth Roberts. Drug-Induced Oxidative Stress and Toxicity. Journal of Toxicology. 2012.

16. B D Banerjee, V Seth, R S Ahmed. Pesticide-induced oxidative stress: perspectives and trends. Reviews on Environmental Health. 2001.

17. Martin Grootveld, Paul B. Addis, and Adam Le Gresley. Editorial: Dietary Lipid Oxidation and Fried Food Toxicology. Frontiers in Nutrition. 2022.

18. Fariheen Aisha Ansari, Riaz Mahmood. Sodium nitrite enhances generation of reactive oxygen species that decrease antioxidant power and inhibit plasma membrane redox system of human erythrocytes. Cell Biology International. 2016.

19. Qian Ge, Zhengjun Wang, Yuwei Wu, et al. High salt diet impairs memory-related synaptic plasticity via increased oxidative stress and suppressed synaptic protein expression. Molecular Nutrition & Food Research. 2017.

20. Kailash Prasad and Indu Dhar. Oxidative Stress as a Mechanism of Added Sugar-Induced Cardiovascular Disease. International Journal of Angiology. 2014.

21. Mustapha Umar Imam, Siti Nor Asma Musa, Nur Hanisah Azmi, Maznah Ismail. Effects of white rice, brown rice and germinated brown rice on antioxidant status of type 2 diabetic rats. International Journal of Molecular Sciences. 2012.

22. Tomoko Monguchi, Tetsuya Hara, Minoru Hasokawa, et al. Excessive intake of trans fatty acid accelerates atherosclerosis through promoting inflammation and oxidative stress in a mouse model of hyperlipidemia. Journal of Cardiology. 2017.

23. Márcio Carocho, Isabel C. F. R. Ferreira, Patricia Morales, and Marina Soković. Antioxidants and Prooxidants: Effects on Health and Aging. Oxidative Medicine and Cellular Longevity. 2018.

24. István Bókkon. Recognition of Functional Roles of Free Radicals. Current Neuropharmacology. 2012.

25. Jaouad Bouayed and Torsten Bohn. Exogenous antioxidants—

Double-edged swords in cellular redox state. Oxidative Medicine and Cellular Longevity. 2010.

26. Graham J. Burton and Eric Jauniaux. Oxidative stress. Best Practice & Research Clinical Obstetrics & Gynaecology. 2011.

27. B N Ames, M K Shigenaga, and T M Hagen. Oxidants, antioxidants, and the degenerative diseases of aging. Proceedings of the National Academy of Sciences. 1993.

28. Marian Valko, Mario Izakovic, Milan Mazur, Christopher J. Rhodes and Joshua Telser. Role of oxygen radicals in DNA damage and cancer incidence. Molecular and Cellular Biochemistry. 2004.

29. Anu Rahal, Amit Kumar, Vivek Singh, et al. Oxidative Stress, Prooxidants, and Antioxidants: The Interplay. BioMed Research International. 2014.

30. Denham Harman, M.D., Ph.D. Aging: A Theory Based on Free Radical and Radiation Chemistry. Journal of Gerontology. 1956.

31. Denham Harman. Free radical theory of aging. Mutation Research/DNAging. 1992.

32. Ergul Belge Kurutas. The importance of antioxidants which play the role in cellular response against oxidative/nitrosative stress: current state. Nutrition Journal. 2016.

33. Henry Jay Forman, Hongqiao Zhang, and Alessandra Rinna. Glutathione: Overview of its protective roles, measurement, and biosynthesis. Molecular Aspects of Medicine. 2009.

34. Christine J Weydert & Joseph J Cullen. Measurement of superoxide dismutase, catalase and glutathione peroxidase in cultured cells and tissue. Nature Protocols. 2009.

35. Francisco Miguel Gutierrez-Mariscal, Antonio Pablo Arenas-de Larriva, Laura Limia-Perez,, et al. Coenzyme Q10 Supplementation for the Reduction of Oxidative Stress: Clinical Implications in the Treatment of Chronic Diseases. MDPI International Journal of Molecular Sciences. 2020.

36. Hiep Nguyen; Vikas Gupta. Alpha-Lipoic Acid. StatPearls. 2021.

37. Premranjan Kumar, Ob Osahon, David B. Vides, et al. Severe Glutathione Deficiency, Oxidative Stress and Oxidant Damage in Adults Hospitalized with COVID-19: Implications for GlyNAC (Glycine and N-Acetylcysteine) Supplementation. MDPI Antioxidants. 2021.

38. Kanti Bhooshan Pandey and Syed Ibrahim Rizv. Plant polyphenols as dietary antioxidants in human health and disease. Oxidative Medicine and Cellular Longevity. 2009.

39. A. N. Panche, A. D. Diwan, and S. R. Chandra. Flavonoids: an overview. Journal of Nutritional Science. 2016.

40. Joanna Fiedor and Květoslava Burda. Potential Role of Carotenoids as Antioxidants in Human Health and Disease. Nutrients. 2014.

41. Mónika Sztretye, Beatrix Dienes, Mónika Gönczi, et al. Astaxanthin: A Potential Mitochondrial-Targeted Antioxidant Treatment in Diseases and with Aging. Oxidative Medicine and Cellular Longevity. 2019.

42. Lavinia Florina Călinoiu and Dan Cristian Vodnar. Whole Grains and Phenolic Acids: A Review on Bioactivity, Functionality, Health Benefits and Bioavailability. MDPI Nutrients. 2018.

43. Maria Celeste Dias, Diana C. G. A. Pinto, and Artur M. S. Silva. Plant Flavonoids: Chemical Characteristics and Biological Activity. Molecules MDPI. 2021.

44. Deanna M. Minich. A Review of the Science of Colorful, Plant-Based Food and Practical Strategies for "Eating the Rainbow." Journal of Nutrition and Metabolism. 2019.

45. Xianli Wu, Gary R. Beecher, Joanne M. Holden, et al. Lipophilic and Hydrophilic Antioxidant Capacities of Common Foods in the United States. Journal of Agricultural and Food Chemistry. 2004.

46. Alexander Yashin, Yakov Yashin, Xiaoyan Xia, and Boris Nemzer. Antioxidant Activity of Spices and Their Impact on Human Health: A Review. Antioxidants. 2017.

47. Meilin Liu, Rolf Wallin, Agneta Wallmon, Tom Saldeen. Mixed tocopherols have a stronger inhibitory effect on lipid peroxidation than alpha-tocopherol alone. Journal of Cardiovascular Pharmacology. 2002.

Tip 2 - Raw Juices: A Health Insurance Policy

1. Vegetables and Fruits. National Institutes of Health (NIH). #PubMed Search.

2. Dagfinn Aune, Edward Giovannucci, Paolo Boffetta, et al. Fruit and vegetable intake and the risk of cardiovascular disease, total cancer and all-cause mortality—a systematic review and dose-response meta-analysis of prospective studies. International Journal of Epidemiology. 2017.

3. Krishan Datt Sharma, Swati Karki, Narayan Singh Thakur, and Surekha Attri. Chemical composition, functional properties and

processing of carrot—a review. Journal of Food Science and Technology. 2011.

4. Yeong Yeh Lee, Askin Erdogan, Satish S C Rao. How to assess regional and whole gut transit time with wireless motility capsule. Journal of Neurogastroenterology and Motility. 2014.

5. Guangwen Tang. Bioconversion of dietary provitamin A carotenoids to vitamin A in humans. The American Journal of Clinical Nutrition. 2010.

6. Emily P. Chea, Michael J. Lopez, Harold Milstein. Vitamin A. StatPearls. 2020.

7. Sergio Martínez Cuesta, Syed Asad Rahman, Nicholas Furnham, and Janet M. Thornton. The Classification and Evolution of Enzyme Function. Biophysical Journal. 2015.

8. Jie Zheng, Yue Zhou, Sha Li, Pei Zhang, et al. Effects and Mechanisms of Fruit and Vegetable Juices on Cardiovascular Diseases. International Journal of Molecule Sciences. 2017.

9. Khalid Rahman. Studies on free radicals, antioxidants, and co-factors. Clinical Interventions in Aging. 2007.

10. Martha E Payne, Susan E Steck, Rebecca R George, David C Steffens. Fruit, vegetable, and antioxidant intakes are lower in older adults with depression. Journal of the Academy of Nutrition and Dietetics. 2012.

11. Kate L. Brookie, Georgia I. Best, and Tamlin S. Conner. Intake of Raw Fruits and Vegetables Is Associated With Better Mental Health Than Intake of Processed Fruits and Vegetables. Frontiers in Psychology. 2018.

12. Qi Dai, MD, PhD, Amy R. Borenstein, PhD, Yougui Wu, PhD, James C. Jackson, PsyD, and Eric B. Larson, MD. Fruit and Vegetable Juices and Alzheimer's Disease: The Kame Project. The American Journal of Medicine. 2006.

13. Susanne M. Henning, Jieping Yang, Paul Shao, et al. Health benefit of vegetable/fruit juice-based diet: Role of microbiome. Scientific Reports. 2017.

14. Kaijian Hou, Zhuo-Xun Wu, Xuan-Yu Chen, et al. Microbiota in health and diseases. Signal Transduction and Targeted Therapy. 2022.

15. 15. Tanveer Ahmad, Maria Cawood, Qumer Iqbal. Phytochemicals in Daucus carota and Their Health Benefits—Review Article. Foods MDPI. 2019.

Tip 3 - Organic Apple Cider Vinegar Remedy

1. Translated by Francis Adams. On Regimen in Acute Diseases By Hippocrates. The Internet Classics Archive at MIT. Written 400 B.C.E.
2. Carol S. Johnston, PhD, RD and Cindy A. Gaas, BS. Vinegar: Medicinal Uses and Antiglycemic Effect. MedGenMed. 2006.
3. Fengge Shen, Jiaxuan Feng, Xinhui Wang, et al. Vinegar Treatment Prevents the Development of Murine Experimental Colitis via Inhibition of Inflammation and Apoptosis. Journal of Agricultural and Food Chemistry. 2016.
4. Singh Akanksha and Sunita Mishra. Study About the Nutritional and Medicinal Properties of Apple Cider Vinegar. Research Gate. 2017.
5. Solaleh Sadat Khezri, Atoosa Saidpour, Nima Hosseinzadeh, Zohreh Amiri. Beneficial effects of Apple Cider Vinegar on weight management, Visceral Adiposity Index and lipid profile in overweight or obese subjects receiving restricted calorie diet: A randomized clinical trial. Journal of Functional Foods. 2018.
6. Tomoo Kondo, Mikiya Kishi, Takashi Fushimi, Shinobu Ugajin, Takayuki Kaga. Vinegar intake reduces body weight, body fat mass, and serum triglyceride levels in obese Japanese subjects. Bioscience, Biotechnology, and Biochemistry. 2009.
7. Ben Hmad Halima, Gara Sonia, Khlifi Sarra, et al. Apple Cider Vinegar Attenuates Oxidative Stress and Reduces the Risk of Obesity in High-Fat-Fed Male Wistar Rats. Journal of Medicinal Food. 2018.
8. Pratul K Agarwal. Enzymes: An integrated view of structure, dynamics and function. Microbial Cell Factories. 2006.
9. Aleksandra Štornik, Barbara Skok, and Janja Trček. Comparison of Cultivable Acetic Acid Bacterial Microbiota in Organic and Conventional Apple Cider Vinegar. Food Technology and Biotechnology. 2016.
10. Judy Gopal, Vimala Anthonydhason, Manikandan Muthu et al. Authenticating apple cider vinegar's home remedy claims: antibacterial, antifungal, antiviral properties and cytotoxicity aspect. Natural Products Research. 2019.
11. E Entani, M Asai, S Tsujihata, Y Tsukamoto, M Ohta. Antibacterial action of vinegar against food-borne pathogenic bacteria including Escherichia coli O157:H7. Journal of Food Protection. 1998.

Tip 4 - Alcohol Health Benefits?

1. Gaetano Di Chiara, MD. Alcohol and Dopamine. Alcohol Health and Research World. 1997.
2. David M. Lovinger, Ph.D. Serotonin's Role in Alcohol's Effects on the Brain. Alcohol Health and Research World. 1997.
3. Susan E Brien, Paul E Ronksley, Barbara J Turner, et al. Effect of alcohol consumption on biological markers associated with risk of coronary heart disease: systematic review and meta-analysis of interventional studies. BMJ. 2011.
4. Gemma Chiva-Blanch and Lina Badimon. Benefits and Risks of Moderate Alcohol Consumption on Cardiovascular Disease: Current Findings and Controversies. Nutrients. 2020.
5. R. Curtis Ellison. Update on the J-shaped Curve for the Relation of Alcohol Intake to Health. Boston University School of Medicine. 2017.
6. Khanh N. Vu, Christie M. Ballantyne, Ron C. Hoogeveen, et al. Causal Role of Alcohol Consumption in an Improved Lipid Profile: The Atherosclerosis Risk in Communities (ARIC) Study. PLOS One. 2016.
7. Kelly A. Volcik, Christie M. Ballantyne, Flavio D. Fuchs, et al. Relationship of Alcohol Consumption and Type of Alcoholic Beverage Consumed With Plasma Lipid Levels: Differences Between Whites and African Americans of the ARIC Study. Annals of Epidemiology. 2008.
8. Zhe Shen, Stefan Munker, Chenyang Wang, et al. Association between alcohol intake, overweight, and serum lipid levels and the risk analysis associated with the development of dyslipidemia. Journal of Clinical Lipidology. 2014.
9. N Nakanishi, H Yoshida, K Nakamura, et al. Influence of alcohol intake on risk for increased low-density lipoprotein cholesterol in middle-aged Japanese men. Alcoholism: Clinical and Experimental Research. 2001.
10. Alexandra Gonçalves, Brian Claggett, Pardeep S. Jhund, et al. Alcohol consumption and risk of heart failure: the Atherosclerosis Risk in Communities Study. European Heart Journal. 2015.
11. H F Hendriks, J Veenstra, E J Velthuis-te Wierik, et al. Effect of moderate dose of alcohol with evening meal on fibrinolytic factors. BMJ. 1994.
12. Edward J Neafsey, Michael A Collins. Moderate alcohol consumption and cognitive risk. Neuropsychiatric Disease and

Treatment. 2011.

13. Kenneth J Mukamal, Lewis H Kuller, Annette L Fitzpatrick, et al. Prospective study of alcohol consumption and risk of dementia in older adults. JAMA. 2003.

14. Kenneth J Mukamal, Lewis H Kuller, Annette L Fitzpatrick, et al. Beneficial effects of low alcohol exposure, but adverse effects of high alcohol intake on glymphatic function. Scientific Reports. 2018.

15. Augusto Di Castelnuovo, ScD; Simona Costanzo, ScD; Vincenzo Bagnardi, ScD, et al. Alcohol Dosing and Total Mortality in Men and Women. JAMA Internal Medicine. 2006.

16. Charles J. Holahan, Kathleen K. Schutte, Penny L. Brennan, et al. Late-Life Alcohol Consumption and 20-Year Mortality. Alcoholism: Clinical and Experimental Research. 2010.

17. Natalia A. Osna, Ph.D., Terrence M. Donohue, Jr., Ph.D., and Kusum K. Kharbanda, Ph.D. Alcoholic Liver Disease: Pathogenesis and Current Management. Alcohol Research. 2017.

18. Francisco D. Rodriguez and Rafael Coveñas. Biochemical Mechanisms Associating Alcohol Use Disorders with Cancers. Cancers MDPI. 2021.

19. R. Nordmann. Alcohol and antioxidant systems. Alcohol and Alcoholism. 1994.

Tip 5 - Healthier Cocktails

1. Amy Mullee, PhD, Dora Romaguera, PhD, Jonathan Pearson-Stuttard, BMBCh, et al. Association Between Soft Drink Consumption and Mortality in 10 European Countries. JAMA Internal Medicine. 2019.

2. Tina M. Saldana, Olga Basso, Rebecca Darden, and Dale P. Sandler. Carbonated Beverages and Chronic Kidney Disease. Epidemiology. 2007.

3. Mani Iyer Prasanth, Bhagavathi Sundaram Sivamaruthi, Chaiyavat Chaiyasut, and Tewin Tencomnao. A Review of the Role of Green Tea (Camellia sinensis) in Antiphotoaging, Stress Resistance, Neuroprotection, and Autophagy. Nutrients. 2019.

4. Sarfraz Ahmed, Siti Amrah Sulaiman, Atif Amin Baig, et al. Honey as a Potential Natural Antioxidant Medicine: An Insight into Its Molecular Mechanisms of Action. Oxidative Medicine and Cellular Longevity. 2018.

5. GG Duthie, MW Pedersen, PT Gardner. The effect of whisky and wine consumption on total phenol content and antioxidant capacity of plasma from healthy volunteers. European Journal of Clinical Nutrition. 1998.

6. En-Qin Xia, Gui-Fang Deng, Ya-Jun Guo, and Hua-Bin Li. Biological Activities of Polyphenols from Grapes. International Journal of Molecular Sciences. 2010.

7. C Baum-Baicker. The psychological benefits of moderate alcohol consumption: a review of the literature. Drug and Alcohol Dependence. 1985.

8. Adrian A. Franke, Robert V. Cooney, Susanne M. Henning, and Laurie J. Custer. Bioavailability and antioxidant effects of orange juice components in humans. Journal of Agricultural and Food Chemistry. 2005.

9. Tasha Barr, Christa Helms, Kathleen Grant, and Ilhem Messaoudi. Opposing Effects of Alcohol on the Immune System. Progress in Neuropsychopharmacology and Biological Psychiatry. 2015.

10. Marcelo Hisano, Homero Bruschini, Antonio Carlos Nicodemo, and Miguel Srougi. Cranberries and lower urinary tract infection prevention. Clinics. 2012.

11. Mary M. Murphy, Leila M. Barraj, and Gail C. Rampersaud. Consumption of grapefruit is associated with higher nutrient intakes and diet quality among adults, and more favorable anthropometrics in women, NHANES 2003–2008. Food & Nutrition Research. 2008.

12. Kirstie Canene-Adams, Jessica K Campbell, Susan Zaripheh, et al. The tomato as a functional food. The Journal of Nutrition. 2005.

13. Moushumi Sur and Shamim S. Mohiuddin. Potassium. StatPearls. 2021.

14. Sudipta Veeramachaneni, Lynne M. Ausman, Sang Woon Choi, et al. High Dose Lycopene Supplementation Increases Hepatic Cytochrome P4502E1 Protein and Inflammation in Alcohol-Fed Rats. The Journal of Nutrition. 2008.

15. Jade Guest, Gilles J. Guillemin, Benjamin Heng, and Ross Grant. Lycopene Pretreatment Ameliorates Acute Ethanol Induced NAD+ Depletion in Human Astroglial Cells. Oxidative Medicine and Cellular Longevity. 2015.

16. Narges Hedayati, Mehri Bemani Naeini, Arash Mohammadinejad, Seyed Ahmad Mohajeri. Beneficial effects of celery (Apium graveolens) on metabolic syndrome: A review of the existing evidences. Phytotherapy Research. 2019.

17. Antonio D Lassaletta, Louis M Chu, Nassrene Y Elmadhun, et al. Cardioprotective effects of red wine and vodka in a model of endothelial dysfunction. Journal of Surgical Research. 2012.

Tip 6 - Red Wine's Potential Health Benefits

1. Luigi Castaldo, Alfonso Narváez, Luana Izzo, et al. Red Wine Consumption and Cardiovascular Health. Molecules. 2019.
2. Attilio Giacosa, Roberto Barale, Luigi Bavaresco, et al. Mediterranean Way of Drinking and Longevity. Critical Reviews in Food Science and Nutrition. 2016.
3. Giacomo Levantesi, RosaMaria Marfisi, Dariush Mozaffarian, et al. Wine consumption and risk of cardiovascular events after myocardial infarction (heart attack): results from the GISSI-Prevenzione trial. International Journal of Cardiology. 2011.
4. T.S. Mohamed Saleem and S. Darbar Basha. Red wine: A drink to your heart. Journal of Cardiovascular Disease Research. 2014.
5. J M Wu, Z R Wang, T C Hsieh, et al. Mechanism of cardioprotection by resveratrol, a phenolic antioxidant present in red wine (Review). International Journal of Molecular Medicine. 2001.
6. D.W. de Lange, P.H. Van Golden, W.L.G. Scholman, et al. Red wine and red wine polyphenolic compounds but not alcohol inhibit ADP-induced platelet aggregation. European Journal of Internal Medicine. 2003.
7. Eleni Pavlidou, Maria Mantzorou, Aristeidis Fasoulas, et al. Wine: An Aspiring Agent in Promoting Longevity and Preventing Chronic Diseases. Diseases MDPI. 2018.
8. Souheila Amor, Pauline Châlons, Virginie Aires and Dominique Delmas. Polyphenol Extracts from Red Wine and Grapevine: Potential Effects on Cancers. Diseases MDPI. 2018.
9. Melissa M. Markoski, Juliano Garavaglia, Aline Oliveira, Jessica Olivaes, and Aline Marcadenti. Molecular Properties of Red Wine Compounds and Cardiometabolic Benefits. Nutrition and Metabolic Insights. 2016.
10. Michelle Micallef, Louise Lexis, and Paul Lewandowski. Red wine consumption increases antioxidant status and decreases oxidative stress in the circulation of both young and old humans. Nutritional Journal. 2007.
11. Jeong-Hyeon Ko, Gautam Sethi, Jae-Young Um, et al. The Role of Resveratrol in Cancer Therapy. International Journal of Molecular Sciences. 2017.

12. S. Renaud, PhD and M. de Lorgeril, MD. Wine, alcohol, platelets, and the French paradox for coronary heart disease. The Lancet Epidemiology. 1992.

13. Giuseppe Lippi, Massimo Franchini, Emmanuel J Favaloro, Giovanni Targher. Moderate red wine consumption and cardiovascular disease risk: beyond the "French paradox." Thieme Seminars in Thrombosis and Hemostasis. 2010.

14. Abdelkader Basli, Stéphanie Soulet, Nassima Chaher, et al. Wine Polyphenols: Potential Agents in Neuroprotection. Oxidative Medicine and Cellular Longevity. 2012.

15. María Isabel Queipo-Ortuño, María Boto-Ordóñez, Mora Murri, et al. Influence of red wine polyphenols and ethanol on the gut microbiota ecology and biochemical biomarkers. The American Journal of Clinical Nutrition. 2012.

16. Victoria Nash, C Senaka Ranadheera, Ekavi N Georgousopoulou, et al. The effects of grape and red wine polyphenols on gut microbiota - A systematic review. Food Research International. 2018.

17. Carly C Barron, Jessy Moore, Theodoros Tsakiridis, et al. Inhibition of human lung cancer cell proliferation and survival by wine. 2014.

18. Jing Duan, Ji-Cheng Zhan, Gui-Zhen WangThe red wine component ellagic acid induces autophagy and exhibits anti-lung cancer activity in vitro and in vivo. Journal of Cellular and Molecular Medicine. 2018.

19. Viktoria Schwarz, MD, Katrin Bachelier, MD, Stephan H. Schirmer, MD, PhD, et al. Red Wine Prevents the Acute Negative Vascular Effects of Smoking. The American Journal of Medicine. 2016.

20. Adelaida Esteban-Fernández, Irene Zorraquín-Peña, Maria D. Ferrer, et al. Inhibition of Oral Pathogens Adhesion to Human Gingival Fibroblasts by Wine Polyphenols Alone and in Combination with an Oral Probiotic. Journal of Agricultural and Food Chemistry. 2018.

21. Daniela Fracassetti, Ileana Vigentini, Alfredo Fabrizio Francesco Lo Faro, et al. Assessment of Tryptophan, Tryptophan Ethylester, and Melatonin Derivatives in Red Wine by SPE-HPLC-FL and SPE-HPLC-MS Methods. Foods MDPI. 2019.

Tip 7 - Beer vs. Wine

1. Julia Wilhelm, Helge Frieling, Thomas Hillemacher, et al. Hippo-

campal volume loss in patients with alcoholism is influenced by the consumed type of alcoholic beverage. Alcohol and Alcoholism. 2008.

2. Rima Obeid, Wolfgang Herrmann. Mechanisms of homocysteine neurotoxicity in neurodegenerative diseases with special reference to dementia. FEBS Letters. 2006.

3. Weiping Fu, Brian S Conklin, Peter H Lin, et al. Red wine prevents homocysteine-induced endothelial dysfunction in porcine coronary arteries. Journal of Surgical Research. 2003.

4. Demosthenes B Panagiotakos, Georgia-Maria Kouli, Emmanuela Magriplis, et al. Beer, wine consumption, and 10-year CVD incidence: the ATTICA study. European Journal of Clinical Nutrition. 2019.

5. Chuan-Hao Jiang, Tao-Li Sun, Da-Xiong Xiang, et al. Anticancer Activity and Mechanism of Xanthohumol: A Prenylated Flavonoid From Hops (Humulus lupulus L.). 2018.

6. V. Neveu, J. Perez-Jiménez, F. Vos, et al. Phenol-Explorer: an online comprehensive database on polyphenol contents in foods. Database: The Journal of Biological Databases and Curation. 2010.

7. Mar Quesada-Molina, Araceli Muñoz-Garach, Francisco J. Tinahones, and Isabel Moreno-Indias. A New Perspective on the Health Benefits of Moderate Beer Consumption: Involvement of the Gut Microbiota. Metabolites MDPI. 2019.

8. Victoria Nash, C Senaka Ranadheera, Ekavi N Georgousopoulou, et al. The effects of grape and red wine polyphenols on gut microbiota - A systematic review. Food Research International. 2018.

9. Teresa Padro, Natàlia Muñoz-García, Gemma Vilahur, et al. Moderate Beer Intake and Cardiovascular Health in Overweight Individuals. Nutrients MDPI. 2018.

10. Dániel Koren, Szilárd Kun, Beáta Hegyesné Vecseri, and Gabriella Kun-Farkas. Study of antioxidant activity during the malting and brewing process. Journal of Food Science and Technology. 2019.

11. Troy R Casey, Charles W Bamforth. Silicon in beer and brewing. The Journal of the Science of Food and Agriculture . 2010.

12. R. Jugdaohsingh. Silicon and Bone Health. The Journal of Nutrition, Health & Aging. 2009.

13. Sara Arranz, Gemma Chiva-Blanch, Palmira Valderas-Martínez, et al. Wine, Beer, Alcohol and Polyphenols on Cardiovascular Disease and Cancer. Nutrients MDPI. 2012.

Tip 8 - Health Concerns with Drinking Alcohol on Empty Stomach

1. Alex Paton. Alcohol in the body. BMJ. 2005.
2. Murray Epstein, M.D. Alcohol's Impact on Kidney Function. Alcohol Healthy and Research World. 1997.
3. Shoukat Ali Samjo, Zaigham Abbas, Muhammad Asim, and Kanwal Tahir. The Pattern of Alcohol Consumption and the Severity of Alcohol-related Liver Disease in Patients Visiting the Liver Clinic. Cureus. 2020.
4. Detlef Schuppan and Nezam H. Afdhal. Liver Cirrhosis. The Lancet. 2008.
5. Alan A Jackson. Nutrition and Liver Health. Digestive Diseases. 2017.
6. Saverio Stranges, Tiejian Wu, Joan M. Dorn, et al. Relationship of Alcohol Drinking Pattern to Risk of Hypertension. Hypertension. 2004.

Tip 9 - Potential Problems with Drinking Beer (or Anything) Out of Aluminum Cans

1. Polymer Coating. ScienceDirect. 2015.
2. Microcracks. ScienceDirect. 2021.
3. Hanns Hippius, MD and Gabriele Neundörfer, MD. The discovery of Alzheimer's disease. Dialogues in Clinical Neuroscience. 2003.
4. Lucija Tomljenovic, PHD. Aluminum and Alzheimer's Disease: After a Century of Controversy, Is there a Plausible Link? Journal of Alzheimer's Disease Reports. 2011.
5. Masahiro Kawahara and Midori Kato-Negishi. Link between Aluminum and the Pathogenesis of Alzheimer's Disease: The Integration of the Aluminum and Amyloid Cascade Hypotheses. International Journal of Alzheimer's Disease. 2011.
6. Ikechukwu Onyebuchi Igbokwe, Ephraim Igwenagu, and Nanacha Afifi Igbokwe. Aluminium toxicosis: a review of toxic actions and effects. Interdisciplinary Toxicology. 2019.
7. Virginie Rondeau, Hélène Jacqmin-Gadda, Daniel Commenges, et al. Aluminum and Silica in Drinking Water and the Risk of Alzheimer's Disease or Cognitive Decline: Findings From 15-Year Follow-up of the PAQUID Cohort. American Journal of Epidemiology. 2008.

8. Ravin Jugdaohsingh, David M Reffitt, Claire Oldham, et al. Oligomeric but not monomeric silica prevents aluminum absorption in humans. The American Journal of Clinical Nutrition. 2000.

9. Fatma M El-Demerdash. Antioxidant effect of vitamin E and selenium on lipid peroxidation, enzyme activities and biochemical parameters in rats exposed to aluminum. Journal of Trace Elements in Medicine and Biology. 2004.

10. David Banji, Otilia J. F. Banji, and Kavati Srinivas. Neuroprotective Effect of Turmeric Extract in Combination with Its Essential Oil and Enhanced Brain Bioavailability in an Animal Model. BioMed Research International. 2021.

11. Wei Bao, Buyun Liu, Shuang Rong, Susie Y Dai, et al. Association Between Bisphenol A Exposure and Risk of All-Cause and Cause-Specific Mortality in US Adults. JAMA Network Open. 2020.

12. Elisabeth Schirmer, Stefan Schuster & Peter Machnik. Bisphenols exert detrimental effects on neuronal signaling in mature vertebrate brains. Nature Communications Biology. 2021.

13. Melanie H Jacobson, Miriam Woodward, Wei Bao, Buyun Liu, Leonardo Trasande. Urinary Bisphenols and Obesity Prevalence Among U.S. Children and Adolescents. Journal of the Endocrine Society. 2019.

14. Melissa Ferguson, Ilka Lorenzen-Schmidt & W. Glen Pyle. Bisphenol S rapidly depresses heart function through estrogen receptor-β and decreases phospholamban phosphorylation in a sex-dependent manner. Scientific Reports. 2019.

15. Shehreen Amjad, Md Saidur Rahman, and Myung-Geol Pang. Role of Antioxidants in Alleviating Bisphenol A Toxicity. Biomolecules MDPA. 2020.

16. Hiral Suthar, R J Verma, Saumya Patel, Y T Jasrai. Green tea potentially ameliorates bisphenol a-induced oxidative stress: an in vitro and in silico study. Biochemistry Research International. 2014.

Tip 10 - Hangover Prevention and Recovery Remedies

1. Jiajing Wang, Leping Jiang, Hanlong Sun. Early evidence for beer drinking in a 9000-year-old platform mound in southern China. PLOS ONE. 2021.

2. Jeri W Nieves, Carmelo Formica, Jamie Ruffing, et al. Males have

larger skeletal size and bone mass than females, despite comparable body size. Journal of Bone and Mineral Research. 2009.

3. Shweta Akhouri; James Kuhn; Edward J. Newton. Wernicke-Korsakoff Syndrome. StatPearls. 2022.

4. Wei Zhong, Zhanxiang Zhou. Sealing the Leaky Gut Represents a Beneficial Mechanism of Zinc Intervention for Alcoholic Liver Disease. 3.1 Physiological Functions of Zinc. Dietary Interventions in Gastrointestinal Diseases. 2019.

5. Isha Shrimanker and Sandeep Bhattarai. Electrolytes. StatPearls. 2020.

6. C J Peter Eriksson, Markus Metsälä, Tommi Möykkynen, et al. L-Cysteine Containing Vitamin Supplement Which Prevents or Alleviates Alcohol-related Hangover Symptoms: Nausea, Headache, Stress and Anxiety. Alcohol and Alcoholism. 2020.

7. Hollis C Karoly, Courtney J Stevens, Rachel E Thayer, et al. Aerobic exercise moderates the effect of heavy alcohol consumption on white matter damage. Alcoholism: Clinical and Experimental Research. 2013.

Tip 11 - Milk "Liver Helper" Thistle

1. Arjun Kalra; Ekrem Yetiskul; Chase J. Wehrle; Faiz Tuma. Physiology, Liver. StatPearls. 2021.

2. Anan Abu Rmilah, Wei Zhou, Erek Nelson, et al. Understanding the marvels behind liver regeneration. WIREs Developmental Biology. 2019.

3. Ted George O. Achufusi; Raj K. Patel. Milk Thistle. StatPearls. 2020.

4. Abby B Siegel and Justin Stebbing. Milk thistle: early seeds of potential. The Lancet Oncology. 2013.

5. Nancy Vargas-Mendoza, Eduardo Madrigal-Santillán, Ángel Morales-González, et al. Hepatoprotective effect of silymarin. World Journal of Hepatology. 2014.

6. Anupom Borah, Rajib Paul, Sabanum Choudhury, Amarendranath Choudhury, et al. Neuroprotective Potential of Silymarin against CNS Disorders: Insight into the Pathways and Molecular Mechanisms of Action. CNS Neuroscience & Therapeutics. 2013.

7. Mariapia Vairetti, Laura Giuseppina Di Pasqua, Marta Cagna, et al. Changes in Glutathione Content in Liver Diseases: An

Update. MDPI Antioxidants. 2021.

8. Anton Gillessen and Hartmut H.-J. Schmidt. Silymarin as Supportive Treatment in Liver Diseases: A Narrative Review. Springer Advances in Therapy. 2020.

Tip 12 - Heartburn Remedy

1. Carolyn Newberry and Kristle Lynch. The role of diet in the development and management of gastroesophageal reflux disease: why we feel the burn. Journal of Thoracic Disease. 2019.

2. Catiele Antunes, Abdul Aleem and Sean A. Curtis. Gastroesophageal Reflux Disease. StatPearls. 2021.

3. Ryan D. Rosen and Ryan Winters. Physiology, Lower Esophageal Sphincter. StatPearls. 2021.

4. Gianluca Ianiro, Silvia Pecere, Valentina Giorgio, et al. Digestive Enzyme Supplementation in Gastrointestinal Diseases. Current Drug Metabolism. 2016.

Tip 13 - Naturally Getting "The Red Out"

1. Michael H. Goldstein, Fabiana Q. Silva, Nysha Blender, et al. Ocular benzalkonium chloride exposure: problems and solutions. Nature Eye. 2022.

2. Claire Gilbert. The eye signs of vitamin A deficiency. 2013.

3. Sadaharu Miyazono, Tomoki Isayama, François C. Delori, and Clint L. Makino. Vitamin A activates rhodopsin and sensitizes it to ultraviolet light. Visual Neuroscience. 2011.

4. Rosie Gilbert, Tunde Peto, Imre Lengyel, Eszter Emri. Zinc Nutrition and Inflammation in the Aging Retina. 2019.

5. Yu-Ping Jia, Lei Sun, He-Shui Yu, et al. The Pharmacological Effects of Lutein and Zeaxanthin on Visual Disorders and Cognition Diseases. Molecules MDPI. 2017.

6. Helen M Rasmussen and Elizabeth J Johnson. Nutrients for the aging eye. Clinical Interventions in Aging. 2013.

Tip 14 - Overcoming Baggy Dark Circles

1. T M Wolever. The glycemic index. World Rev Nutr Diet. 1990.

2. Silke K. Schagen, Vasiliki A. Zampeli, Evgenia Makrantonaki, and Christos C. Zouboulis. Discovering the link between nutrition and skin aging. Dermato-Endocrinology. 2012.

3. Britta De Pessemier, Lynda Grine, Melanie Debaere, et al. Gut–Skin Axis: Current Knowledge of the Interrelationship between Microbial Dysbiosis and Skin Conditions. Microorganisms. 2021.

4. Sang Eun Lee and Seung Hun Lee. Skin Barrier and Calcium. Annals of Dermatology. 2018.

5. Pumori Saokar Telang. Vitamin C in dermatology. Indian Dermatology Online Journal. 2013.

6. Juliet M. Pullar, Anitra C. Carr, and Margreet C. M. Vissers. The Roles of Vitamin C in Skin Health. Nutrients MDPI. 2017.

7. K R Martin. The chemistry of silica and its potential health benefits. The journal of nutrition, health & aging. 2007.

8. James J DiNicolantonio, Jaikrit Bhutani, and James H O'Keefe. The health benefits of vitamin K. Open Heart. 2015.

9. Paraskevi Gkogkolou and Markus Böhm. Advanced glycation end products: Key players in skin aging? Dermato-Endocrinology. 2012.

10. L Packer, H J Tritschler, K Wessel. Neuroprotection by the metabolic antioxidant alpha-lipoic acid. Free Radical Biology and Medicine. 1997.

11. Víctor Manuel Mendoza-Núñez, Beatriz Isabel García-Martínez, Juana Rosado-Pérez, et al. The Effect of 600 mg Alpha-lipoic Acid Supplementation on Oxidative Stress, Inflammation, and RAGE in Older Adults with Type 2 Diabetes Mellitus. Oxidative Medicine and Cellular Longevity. 2019.

12. H. Younus. Therapeutic potentials of superoxide dismutase. IJHS. 2018.

Tip 15 - Naturally Relieving Coughs and Cottonmouth

1. Mandy J. Croyle, Jonathan M. Lehman, Amber K. O'Connor, et al. Role of epidermal primary cilia in the homeostasis of skin and hair follicles. Development. 2011.

Tip 16 - Apples Keep the Lung Doctor Away

1. Barbara K Butland Ann M Fehily, Peter C Elwood. Diet, lung

function, and lung function decline in a cohort of 2512 middle aged men. Thorax. 2000.

2. Yao Li, Jiaying Yao, Chunyan Han, Jiaxin Yang, et al. Quercetin, Inflammation and Immunity. 2016.

3. Dengyu Yang, Tiancheng Wang, Miao Long, Peng Li. Quercetin: Its Main Pharmacological Activity and Potential Application in Clinical Medicine. Oxidative Medicine and Cellular Longevity. 2020.

4. Tram Kim Lam, Melissa Rotunno, Jay H. Lubin, et al. Dietary quercetin, quercetin-gene interaction, metabolic gene expression in lung tissue and lung cancer risk. Carcinogenesis. 2010.

5. Elizabeth A. Townsend and Charles W. Emala, Sr. Quercetin acutely relaxes airway smooth muscle and potentiates β-agonist-induced relaxation via dual phosphodiesterase inhibition of PLCβ and PDE4. American Journal of Physiology. 2013.

6. Jiri Mlcek, Tunde Jurikova, Sona Skrovankova, Jiri Sochor. Quercetin and Its Anti-Allergic Immune Response. Molecules MDPI. 2016.

7. Abigail J. Larson, J. David Symons, and Thunder Jalili. Therapeutic Potential of Quercetin to Decrease Blood Pressure: Review of Efficacy and Mechanisms. Advances in Nutrition. 2012.

8. Josephine Kschonsek, Theresa Wolfram, Annette Stöckl, and Volker Böhm. Polyphenolic Compounds Analysis of Old and New Apple Cultivars and Contribution of Polyphenolic Profile to the In Vitro Antioxidant Capacity. Antioxidants MDPI. 2018.

9. Corrine Hanson, Elizabeth Lyden, Stephen Rennard, et al. The Relationship between Dietary Fiber Intake and Lung Function in the National Health and Nutrition Examination Surveys. Annals of the American Thoracic. 2016.

10. USDA Pesticide Data Program (PDP). Agricultural Marketing Service. 2022.

11. Birgit Wassermann, Henry Müller, and Gabriele Berg. An Apple a Day: Which Bacteria Do We Eat With Organic and Conventional Apples? Frontiers in Microbiology. 2019.

Tip 17 - Fruits and Vegetables for Smokers and Ex-Smokers

1. Radoslav Böhm, Antonín Sedlák, Martin Bulko, Karol Holý. LUNG REGENERATION IN ABSTAINING SMOKERS. Radiation Protection Dosimetry. 2019.

2. Kenichi Yoshida, Kate H. C. Gowers, Henry Lee-Six, et al. Tobacco smoking and somatic mutations in human bronchial epithelium. Nature. 2020.

3. F. L. Büchner, H. B. Bueno-de-Mesquita, J. Linseisen, et al. Fruits and vegetables consumption and the risk of histological subtypes of lung cancer in the European Prospective Investigation into Cancer and Nutrition (EPIC). Springer Cancer Causes & Control. 2009.

4. Martine Shareck, Marie-Claude Rousseau, Anita Koushik, et al. Inverse Association between Dietary Intake of Selected Carotenoids and Vitamin C and Risk of Lung Cancer. Frontiers in Oncology. 2017.

5. J P Eiserich, A van der Vliet, G J Handelman, B Halliwell, and C E Cross. Dietary antioxidants and cigarette smoke-induced biomolecular damage: a complex interaction. The American Journal of Clinical Nutrition. 1995.

6. I Rahman and W MacNee. Oxidant/antioxidant imbalance in smokers and chronic obstructive pulmonary disease (COPD). Thorax. 1996.

7. L. Watson, B. Margetts, P. Howarth, M. Dorward, R. Thompson, P. Little. The association between diet and chronic obstructive pulmonary disease in subjects selected from general practice. European Respiratory Journal. 2002.

8. Haidong Kan, June Stevens, Gerardo Heiss, et al. Dietary fiber, lung function, and chronic obstructive pulmonary disease in the Atherosclerosis Risk in Communities (ARIC) Study. American Journal of Epidemiology. 2008.

9. Vanessa Garcia-Larsen, James F. Potts, Ernst Omenaas, et al. Dietary antioxidants and 10-year lung function decline in adults from the ECRHS survey. European Respiratory Journal. 2017.

10. Virginia Worthington, M.S., Sc.D., C.N.S. Nutritional Quality of Organic Versus Conventional Fruits, Vegetables, and Grains. The Journal of Alternative and Complementary Medicine. 2001.

Tip 18 - Vitamins for Smokers and Ex-Smokers

1. A Catharine Ross. Vitamin A and retinoic acid in T cell-related immunity. The American Journal of Clinical Nutrition. 2012.

2. H.K. Biesalski and D. Nohr. Importance of vitamin-A for lung function and development. Molecular Aspects of Medicine. 2003.

References

3. Ting Li, Agostino Molteni, Predrag Latkovich, et al. Vitamin A Depletion Induced by Cigarette Smoke Is Associated with the Development of Emphysema in Rats. The Journal of Nutrition. 2003.

4. Fumi Hirayama, Andy H. Lee, Colin W. Binns, et al. Do vegetables and fruits reduce the risk of chronic obstructive pulmonary disease (COPD)? A case–control study in Japan. Preventive Medicine. 2009.

5. Jazmine M. Olson; Muhammad Atif Ameer; Amandeep Goyal. Vitamin A Toxicity. StatPearls. 2021.

6. L A Sargeant, A Jaeckel, N J Wareham. Interaction of vitamin C with the relation between smoking and obstructive airways disease in EPIC Norfolk. European Prospective Investigation into Cancer and Nutrition. European Respiratory Journal. 2000.

7. Jie Luo, Li Shen & Di Zheng. Association between vitamin C intake and lung cancer: a dose-response meta-analysis. Scientific Reports. 2014.

8. Sanaappa Virupaxappa Kashinakunti, Pampareddy Kollur, Gurupadappa Shantappa Kallaganada, et al. Comparative study of serum MDA and vitamin C levels in non-smokers, chronic smokers and chronic smokers with acute myocardial infarction in men. Journal of Research in Medical Sciences. 2011.

9. Jane Higdon, Ph.D., Victoria J. Drake, Ph.D., Giana Angelo, Ph.D., et al. Vitamin C. Oregon State University, Linus Pauling Institute. 2000.

10. Nancy E Lange, David Sparrow, Pantel Vokonas, Augusto A Litonjua. Vitamin D Deficiency, Smoking, and Lung Function in the Normative Aging Study. 2012.

11. Rosemary Norton and Maria A. O'Connell. Vitamin D: Potential in the Prevention and Treatment of Lung Cancer. Analogs in Cancer Prevention and Therapy. 2011.

12. Xin Zheng, Nini Qu, Lina Wang, et al. Effect of Vitamin D3 on Lung Damage Induced by Cigarette Smoke in Mice. Open Medicine. 2019.

13. Edgar R. MillerIII, Lawrence J. Appel, Long Jiang and Terence H. Risby. Association Between Cigarette Smoking and Lipid Peroxidation in a Controlled Feeding Study. Circulation. 1997.

14. Hans M.G. Princen, Wim van Duyvenvoorde, Rien Buytenhek, et al. Supplementation With Low Doses of Vitamin E Protects LDL From Lipid Peroxidation in Men and Women. Arteriosclerosis, Thrombosis, and Vascular Biology. 1995.

15. Jiaqi Huang, Stephanie J Weinstein, Kai Yu, et al. A Prospective Study of Serum Vitamin E and 28-Year Risk of Lung Cancer. Journal of the National Cancer Institute. 2019.

16. Richard S. Bruno and Maret G. Traber. Cigarette Smoke Alters Human Vitamin E Requirements. The Journal of Nutrition. 2005.

17. Guohan Chen, Jinyi Wang, Xuan Hong, Zhengjun Chai, and Qinchuan Li. Dietary vitamin E intake could reduce the risk of lung cancer: evidence from a meta-analysis. International Journal of Clinical and Experimental Medicine. 2015.

18. Erin Diane Lewis, Simin Nikbin Meydani, Dayong Wu. Regulatory role of vitamin E in the immune system and inflammation. IUBMB Life. 2018.

19. Chandan K. Sen, Savita Khanna, Cameron Rink, and Sashwati Roy. Tocotrienols: The Emerging Face of Natural Vitamin E. Vitamins & Hormones. 2007.

Tip 19 - The Antioxidant Powers of Grape Seed "Youth" Extract

1. Grape Seed Extract. National Institutes of Health (NIH). #PubMed Search.

2. Abdur Rauf, Muhammad Imran, Tareq Abu-Izneid, et al. Proanthocyanidins: A comprehensive review. Biomedicine & Pharmacotherapy. 2019.

3. Kequan Zhou and Julian J. Raffoul. Potential Anticancer Properties of Grape Antioxidants. Journal of Oncology Hindawi. 2012.

4. John Shi, Jianmel Yu, Joseph E Pohorly, Yukio Kakuda. Polyphenolics in grape seeds-biochemistry and functionality. Journal of Medicinal Food. 2003.

5. Bo Han, Jason Jaurequi, Bao Wei Tang, Marcel E Nimni. Proanthocyanidin: a natural crosslinking reagent for stabilizing collagen matrices. Journal of Biomedical Materials Research. 2003.

6. H R Tang, A D Covington, R A Hancock. Structure-activity relationships in the hydrophobic interactions of polyphenols with cellulose and collagen. Biopolymers. 2003.

7. Aditi Sinha, Nasim Nosoudi, Naren Vyavahare. Elasto-regenerative properties of polyphenols. Biochemical and Biophysical Research Communications. 2014.

8. Lakna. Difference Between Collagen and Elastin. PEDIAA. 2017.

9. Y. Liu, V. Dusevich, and Y. Wang. Proanthocyanidins Rapidly Stabilize the Demineralized Dentin Layer. Journal of Dental Research. 2013.

10. Rani Samyukta Gajjela, R. Kalyan Satish, Girija S. Sajjan, et al. Comparative evaluation of chlorhexidine, grape seed extract, riboflavin/chitosan modification on microtensile bond strength of composite resin to dentin after polymerase chain reaction thermocycling: An in vitro study. Indian Journal of Conservative Dentistry. 2017.

11. Haili Zhang, MM, Shuang Liu, MM, Lan Li, BD, et al. The impact of grape seed extract treatment on blood pressure changes. Medicine. 2016.

12. Ai-Hong Cao, Jian Wang, Hai-Qing Gao, Ping Zhang, and Jie Qiu. Beneficial clinical effects of grape seed proanthocyanidin extract (GSPE) on the progression of carotid atherosclerotic plaques. Journal of Geriatric Cardiology. 2015.

13. Safwen Kadri, Mohamed El Ayed, Pascal Cosette et al. Neuroprotective effect of grape seed extract on brain ischemia: a proteomic approach. Metabolic Brain Disease. 2019.

14. Dae Young Yoo, Woosuk Kim, Ki-Yeon Yoo, et al. Grape seed extract enhances neurogenesis in the hippocampal dentate gyrus in C57BL/6 mice. Phytotherapy Research Wiley. 2011.

15. S Asha Devi, B K Sagar Chandrasekar, K R Manjula, N Ishii. Grape seed proanthocyanidin lowers brain oxidative stress in adult and middle-aged rats. Experimental Gerontology. 2011.

16. Alireza Sarkaki, Maryam Rafieirad, Seyed Ebrahim Hossini, et al. Improvement in Memory and Brain Long-term Potentiation Deficits Due to Permanent Hypoperfusion/Ischemia by Grape Seed Extract in Rats. Iranian Journal of Basic Medical Sciences. 2013.

17. Jun Wang, Lap Ho, Wei Zhao, et al. Grape-Derived Polyphenolics Prevent Aβ Oligomerization and Attenuate Cognitive Deterioration in a Mouse Model of Alzheimer's Disease. Journal of Neuroscience. 2008.

18. Molly Derry, Komal Raina, Rajesh Agarwal, and Chapla Agarwal. Differential Effects of Grape Seed Extract against Human Colorectal Cancer Cell Lines: The Intricate Role of Death Receptors and Mitochondria. Cancer Letters Elsevier. 2013.

19. Oluwadamilola O Olaku, Mary O Ojukwu, Farah Z Zia, Jeffrey D White. The Role of Grape Seed Extract in the Treatment of Chemo/Radiotherapy Induced Toxicity: A Systematic Review of Preclinical Studies. Nutrition and Cancer. 2015.

20. Sangeeta Shrotriya, Gagan Deep, Mallikarjuna Gu, et al. Generation of reactive oxygen species by grape seed extract causes irreparable DNA damage leading to G 2 /M arrest and apoptosis selectively in head and neck squamous cell carcinoma cells. Carcinogenesis. 2012.

21. Debasis Bagchi, Anand Swaroop, Harry G Preuss, Manashi Bagchi. Free radical scavenging, antioxidant and cancer chemoprevention by grape seed proanthocyanidin (GSP): an overview. Mutation Research/Fundamental and Molecular Mechanisms of Mutagenesis. 2014.

22. Marina Reznik. No More Gasping for Air with GSPE. Science Translational Medicine. 2012.

23. Meng-Chun Lu, Mei-Due Yang, Ping-Chun Li, et al. Effect of Oligomeric Proanthocyanidin on the Antioxidant Status and Lung Function of Patients with Chronic Obstructive Pulmonary Disease. In Vivo. 2018.

24. Jenny T. Mao. The Effects of Grape Seed Extract Against Lung Cancer. Albuquerque VA Medical Center. 2014.

25. Jenny T Mao, Qing-Yi Lu, Bingye Xue, et al. A Pilot Study of a Grape Seed Procyanidin Extract for Lung Cancer Chemoprevention. Cancer Prevention Research. 2019.

26. Giovanni B Vigna, Fabrizio Costantini, Giancarlo Aldini, et al. Effect of a standardized grape seed extract on low-density lipoprotein susceptibility to oxidation in heavy smokers. Metabolism. 2003.

27. Miao Liu, Peng Yun, Ying Hu, et al. Effects of Grape Seed Proanthocyanidin Extract on Obesity. Karger Obesity Facts. 2020.

28. Zhipeng Gao, Hua Wu, Kaiqi Zhang, et al. Protective effects of grape seed procyanidin extract on intestinal barrier dysfunction induced by a long-term high-fat diet. Journal of Functional Foods. 2020.

29. Manouchehr Khoshbaten, Akbar Aliasgarzadeh, Koorosh Masnadi, et al. Grape seed extract to improve liver function in patients with nonalcoholic fatty liver change. The Saudi Journal of Gastroenterology. 2010.

30. Gulsum Ozkan, Sukru Ulusoy, Asım Orem, et al. Protective effect of the grape seed proanthocyanidin extract in a rat model of contrast-induced nephropathy. Kidney and Blood Pressure Research. 2012.

31. Jin-Sil Park, Mi-Kyung Park, Hye-Joa Oh, et al. Grape-seed proanthocyanidin extract as suppressors of bone destruction in inflammatory autoimmune arthritis. PLOS ONE. 2012.

32. Sheikh Fayaz Ahmad, Khairy M A Zoheir, Hala E Abdel-Hamied, et al. Grape seed proanthocyanidin extract has potent anti-arthritic effects on collagen-induced arthritis by modifying the T cell balance. International Immunopharmacology. 2013.

33. Atsushi Sano, Shoichi Tokutake, Akihiko Seo. Proanthocyanidin-rich grape seed extract reduces leg swelling in healthy women during prolonged sitting. Journal of the Science of Food and Agriculture. 2013.

34. Ohio State News. Grape Seed Extract Help Speed Up Wound Recovery, Study Suggests. Journal Free Radical Biology and Medicine. 2002.

35. Jose Manuel Silván, Elisa Mingo, Maria Hidalgo, et al. Antibacterial activity of a grape seed extract and its fractions against Campylobacter spp. Food Control. 2013.

36. Aamar Al-Habib, Esmaeil Al-Saleh, Abdel-Majeed Safer, Mohammad Afzal. Bactericidal effect of grape seed extract on methicillin-resistant Staphylococcus aureus (MRSA). The Journal of Toxicological Sciences. 2010.

37. Giovanna Simonetti, Anna Rita Santamaria, Felicia Diodata D'Auria, et al. Evaluation of Anti-Candida Activity of Vitis vinifera L. Seed Extracts Obtained from Wine and Table Cultivars. BioMed Research International. 2014.

38. Santosh K. Katiyar. Grape seed proanthocyanidines and skin cancer prevention: Inhibition of oxidative stress and protection of immune system. Molecular Nutrition & Food Research. 2008.

Tip 20 - Hot Peppers Healthy Buzz

1. Antonella Rosa, Monica Deiana, Viviana Casu, et al. Antioxidant activity of capsinoids. Journal of Agricultural and Food Chemistry. 2002.

2. Jessica O'Neill, Christina Brock, Anne Estrup Olesen, et al. Unravelling the Mystery of Capsaicin: A Tool to Understand and Treat Pain. Pharmacological Reviews. 2012.

3. Dachun Yang, Zhidan Luo, Shuangtao Ma, et al. Activation of TRPV1 (the capsaicin receptor that regulates body temperature) by Dietary Capsaicin Improves Endothelium-Dependent Vasorelaxation and Prevents Hypertension. Cell Metabolism. 2010.

4. Jun Lv, associate professor, Lu Qi, associate professor, Canqing Yu, assistant professor, et al. Consumption of spicy foods and

total and cause specific mortality: population based cohort study. BMJ. 2015.

5. Mustafa Chopan and Benjamin Littenberg. The Association of Hot Red Chili Pepper Consumption and Mortality: A Large Population-Based Cohort Study. PLOS ONE. 2017.

6. Andrew Chang; Alan Rosani; Judy Quick. Capsaicin. StatPearls. NCBI Bookshelf. 2022.

7. Chilli peppers hold promise of preventing liver damage and progression. European Association for the Study of the Liver. 2015.

8. A. Tremblay, H Arguin, and S Panah. Capsaicinoids: a spicy solution to the management of obesity? International Journal of Obesity. 2016.

9. M N Satyanarayana. Capsaicin and gastric ulcers. Critical Reviews in Food Science and Nutrition. 2006.

10. Nicola L Jones, Souheil Shabib, Philip M Sherman. Capsaicin as an inhibitor of the growth of the gastric pathogen Helicobacter pylori. FEMS Microbiology Letters. 1997.

11. Shazia R. Chaudhry; William Gossman. Biochemistry, Endorphin. StatPearls. 2021.

Tip 21 - Sweet Potatoes: A Perfect Munchie Food

1. Sunan Wang, Shaoping Nie, and Fan Zhu. Chemical constituents and health effects of sweet potato. Food Research International. 2016.

2. Fekadu Gurmu, Shimelis Hussein, Mark Laing. The potential of orange-fleshed sweet potato to prevent vitamin A deficiency in Africa. International Journal for Vitamin and Nutrition Research. 2014.

3. Donald Craig Willcox, Giovanni Scapagnini, and Bradley J. Willcox. Healthy aging diets other than the Mediterranean: A Focus on the Okinawan Diet. Mechanisms of Ageing and Development. 2014.

Tip 22 - Garlic and Your Health

1. Leyla Bayan, Peir Hossain Koulivand, and Ali Gorji. Garlic: a review of potential therapeutic effects. Avicenna Journal of Phytomedicine. 2014.

2. Richard S. Rivlin. Historical perspective on the use of garlic. The Journal of Nutrition. 2001.
3. Garlic: National Institutes of Health (NIH). #PubMed Search. 2022.
4. Larry D. Lawson and Scott M. Hunsaker. Allicin Bioavailability and Bioequivalence from Garlic Supplements and Garlic Foods. Nutrients MDPI. 2018.
5. Sonja Krstin, Mansour Sobeh, Markus Santhosh Braun, and Michael Wink. Anti-Parasitic Activities of Allium sativum and Allium cepa against Trypanosoma b. brucei and Leishmania tarentolae. Medicines MDPI. 2018.
6. Limor Horev-Azaria, Shlomit Eliav, Nira Izigov, et al. Allicin up-regulates cellular glutathione level in vascular endothelial cells. European Journal of Nutrition. 2009.
7. J. Songsungkan and Saksit Chanthal. Study of Allicin Extract Chelated with Some Heavy Metals (Cu2+, Co2+ and Pb2+) by Fluorescence Quenching Method and its Antioxidant Activity. Asian Journal of Chemistry. 2014.
8. C.W. Cha. A study on the effect of garlic to the heavy metal poisoning of rat. Journal of Korean Medical Science. 1987
9. Holly L. Nicastro, Sharon A. Ross, and John A. Milne. Garlic and onions: Their cancer prevention properties. Cancer Prevention Research. 2015.
10. S.H. Omar and N.A. Al-Wabel. Organosulfur compounds and possible mechanism of garlic in cancer. Elsevier. 2010.
11. Rodrigo Arreola, Saray Quintero-Fabián, Rocío Ivette López-Roa, et al. Immunomodulation and Anti-Inflammatory Effects of Garlic Compounds. Journal of Immunology. 2015.
12. Zi-Yi Jin, Ming Wu, Ren-Qiang Han, et al. Raw garlic consumption as a protective factor for lung cancer, a population-based case-control study in a Chinese population. Cancer Prevention Research. 2013.
13. Yogeshwer Shukla, Neetu Kalra. Cancer chemoprevention with garlic and its constituents. Cancer Letters ScienceDirect. 2006.
14. Karin Ried, Oliver R Frank, Nigel P Stocks, et al. Effect of garlic on blood pressure: A systematic review and meta-analysis. BMC Cardiovascular Disorders. 2008.
15. Sanjay K Banerjee and Subir K Maulik. Effect of garlic on cardiovascular disorders: a review. Nutrition Journal BMC. 2002.
16. Karin Ried, Catherine Toben, Peter Fakler. Effect of garlic on

serum lipids: an updated meta-analysis. Nutrition Reviews. 2013.

17. Min-Jie Guan, Ning Zhao, Ke-Qin Xie, Tao Zeng. Hepatoprotective effects of garlic against ethanol-induced liver injury: A mini-review. Food and Chemical Toxicology. 2018.

18. Shunming Zhang, Yeqing Gu, Liu Wang, et al. Association between dietary raw garlic intake and newly diagnosed nonalcoholic fatty liver disease: a population-based study. European Journal of Endocrinol. 2019.

Tip 23 - What's the Deal with Red and Processed Meat?

1. Protein and Amino Acids. National Research Council (US) Subcommittee on the Tenth Edition of the Recommended Dietary Allowances. 1989.

2. Susanna C. Larsson, Nicola Orsini. Red Meat and Processed Meat Consumption and All-Cause Mortality: A Meta-Analysis. American Journal of Epidemiology. 2013.

3. Louise Jm Alferink, Jessica C Kiefte-de Jong, Nicole S Erler, et al. Association of dietary macronutrient composition and non-alcoholic fatty liver disease in an ageing population: the Rotterdam Study. BMJ Gut. 2019.

4. Kathryn E Bradbury, Neil Murphy, Timothy J Key. Diet and colorectal cancer in UK Biobank: a prospective study. International Journal of Epidemiology. 2019.

5. Jana J Anderson, Narisa D M Darwis, Daniel F Mackay, et al. Red and processed meat consumption and breast cancer: UK Biobank cohort study and meta-analysis. European Journal of Cancer. 2018.

6. Rashmi Sinha, Yikyung Park, Barry I. Graubard, et al. Meat and Meat-related Compounds and Risk of Prostate Cancer in a Large Prospective Cohort Study in the United States. American Journal of Epidemiology. 2009.

7. Zahra Raisi-Estabragh, Celeste McCracken, Polyxeni Gkontra, et al. Associations of Meat and Fish Consumption With Conventional and Radiomics Cardiovascular Magnetic Resonance Phenotypes in the UK Biobank. Frontiers in Cardiovascular Medicine. 2021.

8. Marta Romeu, Nuria Aranda, Montserrat Giralt, et al. Diet, iron biomarkers and oxidative stress in a representative sample of Mediterranean population. BMC Nutrition Journal. 2013.

9. Jennifer A. Buffa, Kymberleigh A. Romano, Matthew F. Cope-

land, et al. The microbial gbu gene cluster links cardiovascular disease risk associated with red meat consumption to microbiota L-carnitine catabolism. Nature Microbiology. 2021.

10. Zeneng Wang, Nathalie Bergeron, Bruce S Levison, et al. Impact of chronic dietary red meat, white meat, or non-meat protein on trimethylamine N-oxide metabolism and renal excretion in healthy men and women. European Heart Journal. 2018.

11. Vienna E. Brunt, Rachel A. Gioscia-Ryan, Abigail G. Casso, et al. Trimethylamine-N-Oxide Promotes Age-Related Vascular Oxidative Stress and Endothelial Dysfunction in Mice and Healthy Humans. Hypertension. 2020.

12. Zeneng Wang, Adam B. Roberts, Jennifer A. Buffa, et al. Non-lethal Inhibition of Gut Microbial Trimethylamine Production for the Treatment of Atherosclerosis. Cell. 2015.

13. IARC Monographs evaluate consumption of red meat and processed meat. The International Agency for Research on Cancer (IARC). 2015.

14. Yan Zheng, Yanping Li, Ambika Satija, et al. Association of changes in red meat consumption with total and cause specific mortality among US women and men: two prospective cohort studies. BMJ. 2019.

15. Małgorzata Karwowska and Anna Kononiuk. Nitrates/Nitrites in Food—Risk for Nitrosative Stress and Benefits. Antioxidants MDPI. 2020.

16. Susanna C Larsson, Leif Bergkvist, Alicja Wolk. Processed meat consumption, dietary nitrosamines and stomach cancer risk in a cohort of Swedish women. International Journal of Cancer. 2006.

17. Xiu-Juan Xue, Qing Gao, Jian-Hong Qiao, et al. Red and processed meat consumption and the risk of lung cancer: a dose-response meta-analysis of 33 published studies. International Journal of Clinical and Experimental Medicine. 2014.

18. Rui Jiang, David C Paik, John L Hankinson, R Graham Barr. Cured Meat Consumption, Lung Function, and Chronic Obstructive Pulmonary Disease among United States Adults. American Journal of Respiratory and Critical Care Medicine. 2007.

19. Seva G Khambadkone, Zachary A Cordner, Faith Dickerson, et al. Nitrated meat products are associated with mania in humans and altered behavior and brain gene expression in rats. Molecular Psychiatry. 2018.

20. Johanna Mirenda. Celery Powder: What is the purpose of celery powder in organic processing? The Organic Materials Review

Institute (OMRI). 2021.

21. S. R. Tannenbaum. Preventive action of vitamin C on nitrosamine formation. International Journal for Vitamin and Nutrition Research. 1989.

22. Gabriel K. Innes, Keeve E. Nachman, Alison G. Abraham, et al. Contamination of Retail Meat Samples with Multidrug-Resistant Organisms in Relation to Organic and Conventional Production and Processing: A Cross-Sectional Analysis of Data from the United States National Antimicrobial Resistance Monitoring System, 2012–2017. Environmental Health Perspectives. 2021.

23. Chandan Prasad, PhD, Kathleen E. Davis, PhD, RD, Victorine Imrhan, PhD, RD, et al. Advanced Glycation End Products and Risks for Chronic Diseases: Intervening Through Lifestyle Modification. American Journal of Lifestyle Medicine. 2019.

24. Andrew P. Schachat MD, in Ryan's Retina. Diabetic Retinopathy: Genetics and Etiologic Mechanisms. ScienceDirect. 2018.

25. Chemicals in Meat Cooked at High Temperatures and Cancer Risk. NIH National Cancer Institute. 2017.

26. Ewa Grzebyk and Agnieszka Piwowar. Inhibitory actions of selected natural substances on formation of advanced glycation endproducts and advanced oxidation protein products. BMC Complementary and Alternative Medicine. 2016.

27. Youcai Tang, Anping Chen. Curcumin eliminates the effect of advanced glycation end-products (AGEs) on the divergent regulation of gene expression of receptors of AGEs by interrupting leptin signaling. Nature Laboratory Investigation. 2014.

28. Monisha Pradeep, Filmon Kiflezghi Kiflemariam, Eden Tareke. Individual and Combined Effects of Food Components in Attenuating the Formation of Advanced Glycation End Products (AGEs). Food and Nutrition Sciences. 2022.

29. Brush On The Marinade, Hold Off The Cancerous Compounds. University of Arkansas, Food Safety Consortium. 2007.

30. Good news for grilling: Black pepper helps limit cancerous compounds in meat, study shows. Kansas State University. 2017.

Tip 24 - Beating Table Salt's Deadly Addiction

1. Michael J. Morris, Elisa S. Na, and Alan Kim Johnson. Salt craving: The psychobiology of pathogenic sodium intake. Physiology & Behavior. 2008.

2. Mark Derewicz. Your Brain on Salt. UNC Research. 2014.
3. Pasquale Strazzullo, Lanfranco D'Elia, Ngianga-Bakwin Kandala, Francesco P Cappuccio. Salt intake, stroke, and cardiovascular disease: meta-analysis of prospective studies. BMJ. 2009.
4. KY Loh. Know the Common Substance: Table Salt (Sodium chloride, NaCl). Malaysian Family Physician. 2008.
5. William B. Farquhar, PhD, David G. Edwards, PhD, Claudine T. Jurkovitz, MD, and William S. Weintraub, MD. Dietary Sodium and Health: More Than Just Blood Pressure. Journal of the American College of Cardiology. 2015.
6. Katarina Smiljanec and Shannon L. Lennon. Sodium, hypertension, and the gut: does the gut microbiota go salty? American Journal of Physiology. 2019.
7. Katarzyna Jobin, Natascha E Stumpf, Sebastian Schwab, et al. A high-salt diet compromises antibacterial neutrophil responses through hormonal perturbation. Science Translational Medicine. 2020.
8. Hao Ma, Qiaochu Xue, Xuan Wang, et al. Adding salt to foods and hazard of premature mortality. European Heart Journal. 2022.
9. Norm R. C. Campbell and Emma J. Train. A Systematic Review of Fatalities Related to Acute Ingestion of Salt. A Need for Warning Labels? Nutrients MDPI. 2017.
10. Andrea Grillo, Lucia Salvi, Paolo Coruzzi, Paolo Salvi, and Gianfranco Parati. Sodium Intake and Hypertension. Nutrients MDPI. 2019.
11. John E. Hall, PhD. Kidney Dysfunction Mediates Salt-Induced Increases in Blood Pressure. Circulation. 2016.
12. Senthil Selvaraj, Luc Djoussé, Frank G. Aguilar, et al. Association of Estimated Sodium Intake With Adverse Cardiac Structure and Function: From the HyperGEN Study. Journal of the American College of Cardiology. 2017.
13. David G. Edwards and William B. Farquhar. Vascular Effects of Dietary Salt. Current Opinion in Nephrology and Hypertension. 2015.
14. Qian Ge, Zhengjun Wang, Yuwei Wu, et al. High salt diet impairs memory-related synaptic plasticity via increased oxidative stress and suppressed synaptic protein expression. Molecular Nutrition & Food Research. 2017.
15. Giuseppe Faraco, Karin Hochrainer, Steven G. Segarra. et al. Dietary salt promotes cognitive impairment through tau phosphorylation. Nature. 2019.

16. Takuro Kubozono, Masaaki Miyata, Kiyo Ueyama, et al. Acute and chronic effects of smoking on arterial stiffness. Circulation Journal. 2011.

17. Mark F McCarty. Should we restrict chloride rather than sodium? Medical Hypotheses. 2004.

18. Lewis K. Dahl, Martha Heine. Effects of chronic excess salt feeding. Enhanced hypertensogenic effect of sea salt over sodium chloride. Journal of Experimental Medicine. 1961.

19. E. M. Seymour, Andrew A. M. Singer, Maurice R. Bennink, et al. Chronic Intake of a Phytochemical-Enriched Diet Reduces Cardiac Fibrosis and Diastolic Dysfunction Caused by Prolonged Salt-Sensitive Hypertension. Journal of Gerontology. 2008.

20. Qiang Li, Yuanting Cui, Rongbing Jin, et al. Enjoyment of Spicy Flavor Enhances Central Salty-Taste Perception and Reduces Salt Intake and Blood Pressure. Hypertension. 2017.

Tip 25 - Overcoming Sugar Addiction

1. David A. Wiss, Nicole Avena, and Pedro Rada. Sugar Addiction: From Evolution to Revolution. Frontiers in Psychiatry. 2018.

2. James J DiNicolantonio and Amy Berger. Added sugars drive nutrient and energy deficit in obesity: a new paradigm. Open Heart BMJ. 2016.

3. P Mohanty, W Hamouda, R Garg, A Aljada, H Ghanim, P Dandona. Glucose challenge stimulates reactive oxygen species (ROS) generation by leucocytes. The Journal of Clinical Endocrinology & Metabolism. 2000.

4. Quanhe Yang, Zefeng Zhang, Edward W Gregg, et al. Added Sugar Intake and Cardiovascular Diseases Mortality Among US Adults. JAMA Internal Medicine. 2014.

5. Thomas Jensen, Manal F Abdelmalek, Shelby Sullivan, et al. Fructose and sugar: A major mediator of non-alcoholic fatty liver disease. Journal of Hepatology. 2018.

6. Michael Laffin, Robert Fedorak, Aiden Zalasky, et al. A high-sugar diet rapidly enhances susceptibility to colitis via depletion of luminal short-chain fatty acids in mice. Nature Scientific Reports. 2019.

7. Hamid Nasri and Mahmoud Rafieian-Kopaei. Diabetes mellitus and renal failure: Prevention and management. Journal of Research in Medical Sciences. 2015.

8. Anika Knüppel, Martin J. Shipley, Clare H. Llewellyn and Eric J. Brunner. Sugar intake from sweet food and beverages, common mental disorder and depression: prospective findings from the Whitehall II study. Scientific Reports. 2017.

9. H Miao, K Chen, X Yan, F Chen, et al. Sugar in Beverage and the Risk of Incident Dementia, Alzheimer's Disease and Stroke: A Prospective Cohort Study. The Journal of Prevention of Alzheimer's Disease. 2020.

10. Guy E. Townsend II, Weiwei Han, Nathan D. Schwalm III, et al. Dietary sugar silences a colonization factor in a mammalian gut symbiont. PNAS. 2019.

11. SugarScience. How Much Is Too Much? University of California, San Francisco. 2022.

12. Nurbubu T Moldogazieva, Innokenty M Mokhosoev, Tatiana I Mel'nikova, et al. Oxidative Stress and Advanced Lipoxidation and Glycation End Products (ALEs and AGEs) in Aging and Age-Related Diseases. Oxidative Medicine and Cellular Longevity. 2019.

13. H P Nguyen, R Katta. Sugar Sag: Glycation and the Role of Diet in Aging Skin. Skin Therapy Lett. 2015.

14. C. Jeanmaire, L. Danoux, G. Pauly. Glycation during human dermal intrinsic and actinic ageing: an in vivo and in vitro model study. British Journal of Dermatology. 2001.

15. Emel Sahin, Ayse Yesim Göçmen, Hüseyin Koçak, et al.The association of advanced glycation end-products with glutathione status. Annals of Clinical Biochemistry. 2008.

16. 16. Jason Allen and Ryan D. Bradley. Effects of Oral Glutathione Supplementation on Systemic Oxidative Stress Biomarkers in Human Volunteers. Journal of Integrative and Complementary Medicine. 2011.

17. Qinghe Song, Junjun Liu, Liyuan Dong, et al. Novel advances in inhibiting advanced glycation end product formation using natural compounds. Biomedicine & Pharmacotherapy. 2021.

18. Riva Touger-Decker, Cor van Loveren. Sugars and dental caries. The American Journal of Clinical Nutrition. 2003.

19. Amy Lynn Melok, Lee H. Lee, Siti Ayuni Mohamed Yussof, and Tinchun Chu. Green Tea Polyphenol Epigallocatechin-3-Gallate-Stearate Inhibits the Growth of Streptococcus mutans: A Promising New Approach in Caries Prevention. Dentistry Journal MDPI. 2018.

Tip 26 - Kicking the Artificial Sweeteners Non-Nutritive Habit

1. Arbind Kumar Choudhary, Yeong Yeh Lee. Neurophysiological symptoms and aspartame: What is the connection? Nutritional Neuroscience. 2018.

2. Kevin Ouyang, Sunil Nayak, Young Lee, et al. Behavioral effects of Splenda, Equal and sucrose: clues from planarians on sweeteners. Neuroscience Letters. 2016.

3. Charlotte Debras, Eloi Chazelas, Larry Sellem, et al. Artificial sweeteners and risk of cardiovascular diseases: results from the prospective NutriNet-Santé cohort. 2022.

4. Charlotte Debras, Eloi Chazelas, Bernard Srour, et al. Artificial sweeteners and cancer risk: Results from the NutriNet-Santé population-based cohort study. PLOS Medicine. 2022.

5. Matthew P. Pase, Ph.D., Jayandra J. Himali, Ph.D., Alexa S. Beiser, Ph.D., et al. Sugar- and artificially-sweetened beverages and the risks of incident stroke and dementia: A prospective cohort study. Stroke. 2017.

6. Amy Mullee, Dora Romaguera, Jonathan Pearson-Stuttard, et al. Association Between Soft Drink Consumption and Mortality in 10 European Countries. JAMA Internal Medicine. 2019.

7. Michelle Pearlman, Jon Obert, Lisa Casey. The Association Between Artificial Sweeteners and Obesity. Current Gastroenterology Reports. 2017.

8. Georgina Crichton, Ala'a Alkerwi, and Merrrill Elias. Diet Soft Drink Consumption is Associated with the Metabolic Syndrome: A Two Sample Comparison. Nutrients MDPI. 2015.

9. Susan S. Schiffman and H. Troy Nagle. Revisited: Assessing the in vivo data on low/no-calorie sweeteners and the gut microbiota. Food and Chemical Toxicology. 2019.

10. Miriam E. Bocarsly, Elyse S. Powell, Nicole M. Avena, and Bartley G. Hoebel. High-fructose corn syrup causes characteristics of obesity in rats: increased body weight, body fat and triglyceride levels. Pharmacology Biochemistry and Behavior. 2010.

11. William Nseir, Fares Nassar, and Nimer Assy. Soft drinks consumption and nonalcoholic fatty liver disease. World Journal of Gastroenterology. 2010.

12. Jelena Todoric, Giuseppe Di Caro, Saskia Reibe, et al. Fructose stimulated de novo lipogenesis is promoted by inflammation. Nature Metabolism. 2010.

13. Julie Lin and Gary C. Curhan. Associations of Sugar and Arti-

ficially Sweetened Soda with Albuminuria and Kidney Function Decline in Women. Clinical Journal of the American Society of Nephrology. 2011.

14. Richard J Johnson, L Gabriela Sanchez-Lozada, Takahiko Nakagawa. The effect of fructose on renal biology and disease. Journal of the American Society of Nephrology. 2010.

15. Aparna Shil and Havovi Chichger. Artificial Sweeteners Negatively Regulate Pathogenic Characteristics of Two Model Gut Bacteria, E. coli and E. faecalis. International Journal of Molecular Sciences. 2021.

16. Julia Beisner, Anita Gonzalez-Granda, Maryam Basrai, et al. Fructose-Induced Intestinal Microbiota Shift Following Two Types of Short-Term High-Fructose Dietary Phases. Nutrients MDPI. 2020.

Tip 27 - Hold the Canola Oil

1. Erucic Acid. Science Direct Search. 2016.

2. CFR - Code of Federal Regulations Title 21. Rapessed oil. U.S. Food & Drug Administration. 2022.

3. H Vogtmann, R Christian, R T Hardin, D R Clandinin. The effects of high and low erucic acid rapeseed oils in diets for rats. International Journal for Vitamin and Nutrition Research. 1975.

4. M. Saleem and Naveed Ahmad. Characterization of canola oil extracted by different methods using fluorescence spectroscopy. PLOS ONE. 2018.

5. Elisabetta Lauretti & Domenico Praticò. Effect of canola oil consumption on memory, synapse and neuropathology in the triple transgenic mouse model of Alzheimer's disease. Scientific Reports. 2017.

6. Annateresa Papazzo, Xavier A Conlan, Louise Lexis, and Paul A Lewandowski. Differential effects of dietary canola and soybean oil intake on oxidative stress in stroke-prone spontaneously hypertensive rats. Lipids in Health and Disease. 2011.

7. Frank D. Sauer DVM, PhD, Edward R. Farnworth PhD, Jacqueline M.R. Bélanger PhD, et al. Additional vitamin E required in milk replacer diets that contain canola oil. Nutrition Research. 1997.

8. D.J. de Wildt, G.J.A. Speijers. Influence of dietary rapeseed oil and erucic acid upon myocardial performance and hemodynamics in rats. Toxicology and Applied Pharmacology. 1984.

9. Marta Guasch-Ferre, Yanping Li, Walter Willett, et al. Consumption of Olive Oil and Risk of Total and Cause-Specific Mortality Among U.S. Adults. Journal of the American College of Cardiology. 2022.
10. Elisa Mazza, Antonietta Fava, Yvelise Ferro, et al. Effect of the replacement of dietary vegetable oils with a low dose of extra virgin olive oil in the Mediterranean Diet on cognitive functions in the elderly. Journal of Translational Medicine. 2018.

Tip 28 - Soy Health Alert

1. Statement from Susan Mayne, Ph.D., on proposal to revoke health claim that soy protein reduces risk of heart disease. U.S. Food & Drug Administration. 2017.
2. Aneta Popova and Dasha Mihaylova. Antinutrients in Plant-based Foods: A Review. Cross Mark. 2019.
3. Runni Mukherjee, Runu Chakraborty, and Abhishek Dutta. Role of Fermentation in Improving Nutritional Quality of Soybean Meal — A Review. Asian-Australasian Journal of Animal Sciences. 2016.
4. Lisbeth Bohn, Anne S. Meyer, and Søren K. Rasmussen. Phytate: impact on environment and human nutrition. A challenge for molecular breeding. Journal of Zhejiang University SCIENCE B. 2008.
5. J. R. Zhou, E. J. Fordyce, V. Raboy, et al. Reduction of Phytic Acid in Soybean Products Improves Zinc Bioavailability in Rats. The Journal of Nutrition. 1992.
6. Raj Kishor Gupta, Shivraj Singh Gangoliya, and Nand Kumar Singh. Reduction of phytic acid and enhancement of bioavailable micronutrients in food grains. Journal of Food Science and Technology. 2013.
7. Mendel Friedman and David L. Brandon. Nutritional and Health Benefits of Soy Proteins. Journal of Agricultural and Food Chemistry. 2001.
8. Elsa C. Dinsdale and Wendy E. Ward. Early Exposure to Soy Isoflavones and Effects on Reproductive Health: A Review of Human and Animal Studies. Nutrients MDPI. 2010.
9. Medical Memo: Soy and sperm. Harvard Health. 2009.
10. Sergei V. Jargin. Soy and phytoestrogens: possible side effects. GMS German Medical Science. 2014.

11. Daniel R Doerge and Daniel M Sheehan. Goitrogenic and estrogenic activity of soy isoflavones. Environmental Health Perspectives. 2002.
12. K Sukalingam, K Ganesan, S Das, Z C Thent. An insight into the harmful effects of soy protein: A review. La Clinica Terapeutica. 2015.
13. James J DiNicolantonio and James H O'Keefe. Omega-6 vegetable oils as a driver of coronary heart disease: the oxidized linoleic acid hypothesis. Open Heart. 2018.
14. Poonamjot Deol, Jane R. Evans, Joseph Dhahbi, et al. Soybean Oil Is More Obesogenic and Diabetogenic than Coconut Oil and Fructose in Mouse: Potential Role for the Liver. PLOS ONE. 2015.
15. Poonamjot Deol, Elena Kozlova, Matthew Valdez, et al. Dysregulation of Hypothalamic Gene Expression and the Oxytocinergic System by Soybean Oil Diets in Male Mice. Endocrinology. 2020.

Tip 29 - Celery Health

1. Ravin Jugdaohsingh, Abigail I.E. Watson, Liliana D. Pedro, and Jonathan J. Powell. The decrease in silicon concentration of the connective tissues with age in rats is a marker of connective tissue turnover. Bone Elsevier. 2015.
2. Wesam Kooti, MSc and Nahid Daraei, MSc. A Review of the Antioxidant Activity of Celery. The Journal of Evidence-Based Integrative Medicine. 2017.
3. Bokyung Sung, Hae Young Chung, and Nam Deuk Kim. Role of Apigenin in Cancer Prevention via the Induction of Apoptosis and Autophagy. Journal of Cancer Prevention. 2016.
4. Nathalie Pross. Effects of Dehydration on Brain Functioning: A Life-Span Perspective. Annals of Nutrition and Metabolism. 2017.

Tip 30 - Importance of Vitamin B Complex

1. Aparna Sheetal, Vinay Kumar Hiremath, Anand G Patil, et al. Malnutrition and its Oral Outcome – A Review. Journal of Clinical and Diagnostic Research. 2013.
2. Kathleen Mikkelsen, Vasso Apostolopoulos. B Vitamins and

Ageing. Biochemistry and Cell Biology of Ageing. 2019.

3. Julian-Dario Rembe, Carolin Fromm-Dornieden, Ewa Klara Stuermer. Effects of Vitamin B Complex and Vitamin C on Human Skin Cells: Is the Perceived Effect Measurable? Advances in Skin & Wound Care. 2018.

4. Talitha C. Ford, Luke A. Downey, Tamara Simpson, Grace McPhee, Chris Oliver, and Con Stough. The Effect of a High-Dose Vitamin B Multivitamin Supplement on the Relationship between Brain Metabolism and Blood Biomarkers of Oxidative Stress: A Randomized Control Trial. Nutrients MDPI. 2018.

5. Ken Yoshii, Koji Hosomi, Kento Sawane, and Jun Kunisawa. Metabolism of Dietary and Microbial Vitamin B Family in the Regulation of Host Immunity. Frontiers in Nutrition. 2019.

6. Carlos Alberto Calderón-Ospina and Mauricio Orlando Nava-Mesa. B Vitamins in the nervous system: Current knowledge of the biochemical modes of action and synergies of thiamine, pyridoxine, and cobalamin. CNS Neuroscience & Therapeutics. 2020.

7. Victoria J. Drake, Ph.D. Cognitive Function In Depth. Oregon State University. The Linus Pauling Institute Micronutrient Information Center. 2011.

8. Marziyeh Ashoori, Ahmad Saedisomeolia. Riboflavin (vitamin B_2) and oxidative stress: a review. British Journal of Nutrition. 2014.

9. Lauren M Young, Andrew Pipingas, David J White, Sarah Gauci, and Andrew Scholey. A Systematic Review and Meta-Analysis of B Vitamin Supplementation on Depressive Symptoms, Anxiety, and Stress: Effects on Healthy and 'At-Risk' Individuals. Nutrients MDPI. 2019.

10. Karen M. Ryan, Kelly A. Allers, Andrew Harkin, Declan M. McLoughlin. Blood plasma B vitamins in depression and the therapeutic response to electroconvulsive therapy. Brain, Behavior, & Immunity - Health. 2020.

11. S Cook, O M Hess. Homocysteine and B vitamins. Handbook of Experimental Pharmacology. 2005.

12. Katherine L Tucker, Ning Qiao, Tammy Scott, Irwin Rosenberg, Avron Spiro, III. High homocysteine and low B vitamins predict cognitive decline in aging men: the Veterans Affairs Normative Aging Study. The American Journal of Clinical Nutrition. 2005.

13. Salah Gariballa. Testing homocysteine-induced neurotransmitter deficiency, and depression of mood hypothesis in clinical practice. Age and Ageing. 2011.

14. David O. Kennedy. B Vitamins and the Brain: Mechanisms, Dose and Efficacy—A Review. Nutrients MDPI. 2016.
15. Gary E Gibson and John P Blass. Nutrition and Functional Neurochemistry. 1999.

Tip 31 - Health Benefits of Raw Nuts and Seeds

1. Rávila Graziany Machado de Souza, Raquel Machado Schincaglia, Gustavo Duarte Pimentel, and João Felipe Mota. Nuts and Human Health Outcomes: A Systematic Review. Nutrients MDPI. 2017.
2. Richard E Ostlund Jr. Phytosterols and cholesterol metabolism. Current Opinion in Lipidology. 2004.
3. Theodore Lewis; William L. Stone. Biochemistry, Proteins Enzymes. StatPearls. 2021.
4. Sofia C. Lourenço, Margarida Moldão-Martins, and Vítor D. Alves. Antioxidants of Natural Plant Origins: From Sources to Food Industry Applications. Molecules MDPI. 2019.
5. AM Coates, AM Hill, & SY Tan. Nuts and Cardiovascular Disease Prevention. Current Atherosclerosis Reports. 2018.
6. Susanna C Larsson, Nikola Drca, Martin Björck, Magnus Bäck, Alicja Wolk. Nut consumption and incidence of seven cardiovascular disease. Heart. 2018.
7. Ming Li and Z. Shi. A Prospective Association of Nut Consumption with Cognitive Function in Chinese Adults Aged 55+ _ China Health and Nutrition Survey. The journal of nutrition, health & aging. 2019.
8. Narjes Gorji, Reihaneh Moeini, Zahra Memariani. Almond, hazelnut and walnut, three nuts for neuroprotection in Alzheimer's disease: A neuropharmacological review of their bioactive constituents. Pharmacological Research. 2018.
9. Abha Chauhan and Ved Chauhan. Beneficial Effects of Walnuts on Cognition and Brain Health. Nutrients MDPI. 2020.
10. Florence Gignac, Dora Romaguera, Silvia Fernández-Barrés, et al. Maternal nut intake in pregnancy and child neuropsychological development up to 8 years old: a population-based cohort study in Spain. European Journal of Epidemiology. 2019.
11. Chandra L Jackson and Frank B Hu. Long-term associations of nut consumption with body weight and obesity. The American Journal of Clinical Nutrition. 2014.

12. Jaya Kumar, Srijit Das, and Seong Lin Teoh. Dietary Acrylamide and the Risks of Developing Cancer: Facts to Ponder. Frontiers in Nutrition. 2018.
13. Raj Kishor Gupta, Shivraj Singh Gangoliya, and Nand Kumar Singh. Reduction of phytic acid and enhancement of bioavailable micronutrients in food grains. Journal of Food Science and Technology 2013.

Tip 32 - Scoring the Best Bread

1. Dagfinn Aune, NaNa Keum, Edward Giovannucci, et al. Whole grain consumption and risk of cardiovascular disease, cancer, and all cause and cause specific mortality: systematic review and dose-response meta-analysis of prospective studies. BMJ. 2016.
2. Wanshui Yang, Yanan Ma, Yue Liu, et al. Association of Intake of Whole Grains and Dietary Fiber With Risk of Hepatocellular Carcinoma in US Adults. JAMA Oncology. 2019.
3. Parke Wilde, Jennifer L Pomeranz, Lauren J Lizewski, Fang Fang Zhang. Consumer confusion about wholegrain content and healthfulness in product labels: a discrete choice experiment and comprehension assessment. Public Health Nutrition Cambridge. 2020.
4. Wonder Bread. Wikipedia. 2022.
5. Nancy Lee Swanson, Andre Frederick Leu, Jon Abrahamson, Bradley C. Wallet. Genetically engineered crops, glyphosate and the deterioration of health in the United States of America. Research Gate. 2014.
6. Crop desiccation. Wikipedia. 2022.
7. John Peterson Myers, Michael N. Antoniou, Bruce Blumberg, et al. Concerns over use of glyphosate-based herbicides and risks associated with exposures: a consensus statement. Environmental Health. 2016.
8. Anthony Samsel and Stephanie Seneff. Glyphosate, pathways to modern diseases IV: cancer and related pathologies. Journal of Biological Physics and Chemistry. 2015.
9. CFR - Code of Federal Regulations Title 21. U.S. Food & Drug Administration. 2020.
10. A. C. Frazer, J. R. Hickman, H. G. Sammons, M. Sharratt. Studies on the effects of treatment with chlorine dioxide on the properties of wheat flour. III.†—Lipid changes and vitamin content of treated flours. The Journal of the Science of Food and Agricul-

ture. 1956.

11. Vita Giaccone, Gaetano Cammilleri, Vita Di Stefano, et al. First report on the presence of Alloxan in bleached flour by LC-MS/MS method. Journal of Cereal Science. 2017.

12. Imane Song, Oelfah Patel, Eddy Himpe, Christo J F Muller, Luc Bouwens. Beta Cell Mass Restoration in Alloxan-Diabetic Mice Treated with EGF and Gastrin. PLOS ONE. 2015.

13. Peter J. Havel. A scientific review: the role of chromium in insulin resistance. Diabetes Education. 2004.

14. Yuni Choi, Edward Giovannucci, Jung Eun Lee. Glycaemic index and glycaemic load in relation to risk of diabetes-related cancers: a meta-analysis. British Journal of Nutrition. 2012.

15. J Philip Karl, Mohsen Meydani, Junaidah B Barnett, et al. Substituting whole grains for refined grains in a 6-wk randomized trial favorably affects energy-balance metrics in healthy men and postmenopausal women. The American Journal of Clinical Nutrition. 2017.

16. Carmen de la Fuente-Arrillaga, Miguel Angel Martinez-Gonzalez, Itziar Zazpe, et al. Glycemic load, glycemic index, bread and incidence of overweight/obesity in a Mediterranean cohort: the SUN project. BMC Public Health. 2014.

17. Y Kurokawa, A Maekawa, M Takahashi, and Y Hayashi. Toxicity and carcinogenicity of potassium bromate--a new renal carcinogen. Environmental Health Perspectives. 1990.

18. Lavinia Florina Călinoiu and Dan Cristian Vodnar. Whole Grains and Phenolic Acids: A Review on Bioactivity, Functionality, Health Benefits and Bioavailability. MDPI Nutrients. 2018.

Tip 33 - Wheatgrass Juice "Healing" Shots

1. F. Ogutu, S. I. Makori, Christine Wanja Maringa, Daniel Lemtukei, Gertrude Okiko, Susan Luvita. Wheat Grass: A Functional Food. Food Science and Quality Management. 2017.

2. AP Khapre, DM Shere, HW Deshpande. Health and nutritional benefits of wheat grass juice. Advances in Plants & Agriculture Research. 2019.

3. Santosh B Parit, Vishal V Dawkar, Rahul S Tanpure, Sandeep R Pai, Ashok D Chougale. Nutritional Quality and Antioxidant Activity of Wheatgrass (Triticum aestivum) Unwrap by Proteome Profiling and DPPH and FRAP assay. Journal of Food Science. 2018.

4. M. Chauhan. A pilot study on wheat grass juice for its phytochemical, nutritional and therapeutic potential on chronic diseases. International Journal of Chemical Studies. 2014.

5. Masood Shah Khan, Rabea Parveen, Kshipra Mishra, Rajkumar Tulsawani, and Sayeed Ahmad. Chromatographic analysis of wheatgrass extracts. Journal of Pharmacy & BioAllied Sciences. 2015.

6. Rucha Diwakar Gore, Sangeeta Jayant Palaskar, and Anirudha Ratnadeep Bartake. Wheatgrass: Green Blood can Help to Fight Cancer. Journal of Clinical and Diagnostic Research. 2017.

7. Sunil D. Kulkarni, Jai. C. Tilak, R. Acharya, et al. Evaluation of the antioxidant activity of wheatgrass (Triticum aestivum L.) as a function of growth under different conditions. Phytotherapy Research. 2006.

8. Kateřina Vaňková, Ivana Marková, Jana Jašprová, et al. Chlorophyll-Mediated Changes in the Redox Status of Pancreatic Cancer Cells Are Associated with Its Anticancer Effects. Oxidative Medicine and Cellular Longevity. 2018.

9. Erjia Wang and Michael Wink. Chlorophyll enhances oxidative stress tolerance in Caenorhabditis elegans and extends its lifespan. PeerJ. 2016.

Tip 34 - Organic Produce or Bust?

1. Environmental Working Group's (EWG) Shopper's Guide to Pesticides in Produce. 2021.

2. U.S. Centers for Disease Control: Fourth National Report on Human Exposure to Environmental Chemicals. 2009.

3. Polyxeni Nicolopoulou-Stamati, Sotirios Maipas, Chrysanthi Kotampasi, Panagiotis Stamatis, and Luc Hens. Chemical Pesticides and Human Health: The Urgent Need for a New Concept in Agriculture. Frontiers in Public Health. 2016.

4. Y.H. Chiu, M.C. Afeiche, A.J. Gaskins, et al. Fruit and vegetable intake and their pesticide residues in relation to semen quality among men from a fertility clinic. Human Reproduction. 2015.

5. Yu-Han Chiu, MD, ScD, Paige L. Williams, PhD, Matthew W. Gillman, MD, SM, et al. Association Between Pesticide Residue Intake From Consumption of Fruits and Vegetables and Pregnancy Outcomes. JAMA Internal Medicine. 2018.

6. Ondine S von Ehrenstein, Chenxiao Ling, Xin Cui, et al.

Prenatal and infant exposure to ambient pesticides and autism spectrum disorder in children: population based case-control study. BMJ. 2019.

7. Bridget M. Kuehn. Increased Risk of ADHD Associated With Early Exposure to Pesticides, PCBs. JAMA Network. 2010.

8. Carly Hyland, Asa Bradman, Roy Gerona, et al. Organic diet intervention significantly reduces urinary pesticide levels in U.S. children and adults. Environmental Research. 2019.

9. John Fagan, Larry Bohlen, Sharyle Patton, Kendra Klein. Organic diet intervention significantly reduces urinary glyphosate levels in U.S. children and adults. Environmental Research. 2020.

10. Julia Baudry, Karen E Assmann, Mathilde Touvier, et al. Association of Frequency of Organic Food Consumption With Cancer Risk: Findings From the NutriNet-Santé Prospective Cohort Study. JAMA Internal Medicine. 2018.

11. Yong-Moon Mark Park, Alexandra White, Nicole Niehoff, Katie O'Brien, Dale Sandler. Association Between Organic Food Consumption and Breast Cancer Risk: Findings from the Sister Study (P18-038-19). Current Developments in Nutrition. 2019.

12. Virginia Worthington. Nutritional Quality of Organic Versus Conventional Fruits, Vegetables, and Grains. Journal of Integrative and Complementary Medicine. 2004.

13. Marcin Barański, Dominika Srednicka-Tober, Nikolaos Volakakis, et al. Higher antioxidant and lower cadmium concentrations and lower incidence of pesticide residues in organically grown crops: a systematic literature review and meta-analyses. British Journal of Nutrition. 2014.

14. Environmental Working Group's (EWG) Annual Dirty Dozen and Clean Fifteen Shopper's Guild. 2022.

15. Thomas G. Neltner, Neesha R. Kulkarni, Heather M. Alger, et al. Navigating the U.S. Food Additive Regulatory Program. Comprehensive Reviews in Food Science and Food Safety. 2011.

16. Miles McEvoy. Organic 101: What the USDA Organic Label Means. U.S. Department of Agriculture. 2019.

17. Carbon Sequestration. Rodale Institute. 2021.

Tip 35 - Cruciferous Vegetables for Cancer Prevention and Overall Better Health

1. Geert van Poppel, Dorette T. H. Verhoeven, Hans Verhagen, R. Alexandra Goldbohm. Brassica Vegetables and Cancer Prevention. Advances in Nutrition and Cancer. 1999.

2. Asvinidevi Arumugam, Ahmad Faizal Abdull Razis. Apoptosis as a Mechanism of the Cancer Chemopreventive Activity of Glucosinolates: a Review. Asian Pacific Journal of Cancer Prevention. 2018.

3. Adarsh Pal Vig, Geetanjali Rampal, Tarunpreet Singh Thind, Saroj Arora. Bio-protective effects of glucosinolates – A review. Research Gate. 2009.

4. Meike Burow, Barbara Ann Halkier. How does a plant orchestrate defense in time and space? Using glucosinolates in Arabidopsis as case study. Current Opinion in Plant Biology. 2017.

5. Francisco Fuentes, Ximena Paredes-Gonzalez, and Ah-Ng Tony Kong. Dietary Glucosinolates Sulforaphane, Phenethyl Isothiocyanate, Indole-3-Carbinol/3,3'-Diindolylmethane: Anti-Oxidative Stress/Inflammation, Nrf2, Epigenetics/Epigenomics and In Vivo Cancer Chemopreventive Efficacy. Current Pharmacology Reports. 2015.

6. Herbert Tilg. Cruciferous vegetables: prototypic anti-inflammatory food components. Clinical Phytoscience. 2015.

7. Francisco J. Barba, Nooshin Nikmaram, Shahin Roohinejad, Anissa Khelfa, Zhenzhou Zhu, and Mohamed Koubaa. Bioavailability of Glucosinolates and Their Breakdown Products: Impact of Processing. Frontiers in Nutrition. 2016.

8. John D. Clarke, Roderick H. Dashwood, and Emily Ho. Multi-targeted prevention of cancer by sulforaphane. Cancer Letters. 2008.

9. Jane V. Higdon, Barbara Delage, David E. Williams, and Roderick H. Dashwood. Cruciferous Vegetables and Human Cancer Risk: Epidemiologic Evidence and Mechanistic Basis. Pharmacological Research. 2007.

10. Kendra J. Royston, B.S. and Trygve O. Tollefsbol, D.O. Ph.D. The Epigenetic Impact of Cruciferous Vegetables on Cancer Prevention. Current Pharmacology Reports. 2015.

11. Alena Vanduchova, Pavel Anzenbacher, Eva Anzenbacherova. Isothiocyanate from Broccoli, Sulforaphane, and Its Properties. Journal of Medicinal Food. 2019.

12. Eri Kubo, Bhavana Chhunchha, Prerna Singh, Hiroshi Sasaki, Dhirendra P Singh. Sulforaphane reactivates cellular antioxidant defense by inducing Nrf2/ARE/Prdx6 activity during aging and oxidative stress. Scientific Reports. 2017.

13. Xin Jiang, Ye Liu, Lixin Ma, et al. Chemopreventive activity of sulforaphane. Drug Design, Development and Therapy Journal. 2018.

14. Jisung Kim, Siyoung Lee, Bo-Ryoung Choi, et al. Sulforaphane epigenetically enhances neuronal BDNF expression and TrkB signaling pathways. Molecular Nutrition & Food Research. 2016.

15. Sedlak T.W., Nucifora L.G., Koga M., et al. Sulforaphane Augments Glutathione and Influences Brain Metabolites in Human Subjects: A Clinical Pilot Study. Complex Psychiatry. 2017.

16. Leilei Mao, Tuo Yang, Xin Li, et al. Protective effects of sulforaphane in experimental vascular cognitive impairment: Contribution of the Nrf2 pathway. Journal of Cerebral Blood Flow & Metabolism. 2018.

17. Pramod K Dash, Jing Zhao, Sara A Orsi, Min Zhang, Anthony N Moore. Sulforaphane improves cognitive function administered following traumatic brain injury. Neuroscience Letters. 2009.

18. Barbara Licznerska, Wanda Baer-Dubowska. Indole-3-Carbinol and Its Role in Chronic Diseases. Advances in Experimental Medicine and Biology. 2016.

19. Linqiang Ma, Honggui Li, Jinbo Hu, et al. Indole Alleviates Diet-Induced Hepatic Steatosis and Inflammation in a Manner Involving Myeloid Cell 6-Phosphofructo-2-Kinase/Fructose-2,6-Biphosphatase 3. Hepatology. 2020.

20. Kent State University. Indole-3-carbinol inhibition of herpes simplex virus replication. Europe PMC. 2011.

21. Catarina M. Quinzii and Michio Hirano. Coenzyme Q and Mitochondrial Disease. Developmental Disabilities Research Reviews. 2010.

22. Paul S Bernstein, Binxing Li, Preejith P Vachali, et al. Lutein, zeaxanthin, and meso-zeaxanthin: The basic and clinical science underlying carotenoid-based nutritional interventions against ocular disease. Progress in Retinal and Eye Research. 2016.

23. Krystle E Zuniga, Nicholas J Bishop, Alexandria S Turner. Dietary lutein and zeaxanthin are associated with working memory in an older population. Public Health Nutrition. 2020.

24. Mark M. Jones. Heavy-Metal Detoxification Using Sulfur Compounds. Sulfur Reports. 1985.

25. Li Tang, Gary R Zirpoli, Vijayvel Jayaprakash, et al. Cruciferous vegetable intake is inversely associated with lung cancer risk

among smokers: a case-control study. BMC Cancer. 2010.

26. Q J Wu, L Xie, W Zheng, et al. Cruciferous vegetables consumption and the risk of female lung cancer: a prospective study and a meta-analysis. Annals of Oncology. 2013.

27. David G Walters, Philip J Young, Cynthia Agus, et al. Cruciferous vegetable consumption alters the metabolism of the dietary carcinogen 2-amino-1-methyl-6-phenylimidazo[4,5-b]pyridine (PhIP) in humans. Carcinogenesis. 2004.

28. Lilli B Link, John D Potter. Raw versus cooked vegetables and cancer risk. Cancer Epidemiology, Biomarkers & Prevention. 2004.

29. C C Conaway, S M Getahun, L L Liebes, et al. Disposition of glucosinolates and sulforaphane in humans after ingestion of steamed and fresh broccoli. Nutrition and Cancer. 2000.

30. S A McNaughton, G C Marks. Development of a food composition database for the estimation of dietary intakes of glucosinolates, the biologically active constituents of cruciferous vegetables. British Journal of Nutrition. 2003.

31. Gao-feng Yuan, Bo Sun, Jing Yuan & Qiao-mei Wang. Effects of different cooking methods on health-promoting compounds of broccoli. Journal of Zhejiang University SCIENCE B. 2009.

32. F. Vallejo, F. Tomás-Barberán & C. García-Viguera. Glucosinolates and vitamin C content in edible parts of broccoli florets after domestic cooking. European Food Research and Technology. 2002.

33. F Vallejo, FA Tomás-Barberán, C García-Viguera. Phenolic compound contents in edible parts of broccoli inflorescences after domestic cooking. Journal of the Science of Food and Agriculture. 2003.

34. Benedict C. Eke, Norbert N. Jibiri, Evelyn N. Bede, et al. Effect of ingestion of microwaved foods on serum anti-oxidant enzymes and vitamins of albino rats. Journal of Radiation Research and Applied Sciences. 2017.

35. Wook Jin Choi, Jeongseon Kim. Dietary factors and the risk of thyroid cancer: a review. Korean Society of Clinical Nutrition. 2014.

Tip 36 - Lemon Aid

1. Anna Czech, Ewa Zarycka, Dmytro Yanovych, et al. Mineral Content of the Pulp and Peel of Various Citrus Fruit Cultivars.

Biological Trace Element Research. 2019.

2. shahabeddin Bahrani, Seyed, Abdulkarimi, Rahim, sabziyani, Zahra, et al. The comparison of the effect of garlic and lemon juice on blood pressure and comfort in hypertensive patients. EBSCO Publishing. 2020.

3. Ayman M. Mahmoud, Rene J. Hernández Bautista, Mansur A. Sandhu, and Omnia E. Hussein. Beneficial Effects of Citrus Flavonoids on Cardiovascular and Metabolic Health. Oxidative Medicine and Cellular Longevity. 2019.

4. Maya E. Kotas and Ruslan Medzhitov. Homeostasis, Inflammation, and Disease Susceptibility. Cell. 2015.

5. Jens Lykkesfeldt. Vitamin C. Advances in Nutrition. 2014.

6. Free Radicals and Reactive Oxygen. Vivo Pathophysiology Colorado State University.

7. Amit Roy, Shailendra Saraf. Limonoids: overview of significant bioactive triterpenes distributed in plants kingdom. Biological and Pharmaceutical Bulletin. 2006.

8. Soraya Mousavi, Stefan Bereswill, and Markus M. Heimesaat. Immunomodulatory and Antimicrobial Effects of Vitamin C. European Journal of Microbiology and Immunology. 2019.

9. Aida Haddad, Shamim S. Mohiuddin. Biochemistry, Citric Acid Cycle. StatPearls. 2022.

10. Ehigbai I. Oikeh, Ehimwenma S. Omoregie, Faith E. Oviasogie, and Kelly Oriakhi. Phytochemical, antimicrobial, and antioxidant activities of different citrus juice concentrates. Food Science & Nutrition. 2015.

11. Omar M.E. Abdel-Salam, Eman R. Youness, Nadia A. Mohammed, Safaa M. Youssef Morsy, Enayat A. Omara, and Amany A. Sleem. Chapter 16 - Citric Acid an Antioxidant in Liver. The Liver: Oxidative Stress and Dietary Antioxidant. 2018.

12. Kristina L. Penniston, Thomas H. Steele, Stephen Y. Nakada. Lemonade Therapy Increases Urinary Citrate and Urine Volumes in Patients with Recurrent Calcium Oxalate Stone Formation. Urology. 2007.

13. Rosaria Ciriminna, Francesco Meneguzzo, Riccardo Delisi, and Mario Pagliaro. Citric acid: emerging applications of key biotechnology industrial product. BMC Chemistry. 2017.

14. Iliana E. Sweis and Bryan C. Cressey. Potential role of the common food additive manufactured citric acid in eliciting significant inflammatory reactions contributing to serious disease states: A series of four case reports. Toxicology Reports. 2016.

15. Xiaoguang Chen, Qiongxia Lv, Yumei Liu, and Wen Deng. Study on injury effect of food additive citric acid on liver tissue in mice. Cytotechnology. 2014.

16. Tong Zhou, Yu-Jie Zhang, Dong-Ping Xu, et al. Protective Effects of Lemon Juice on Alcohol-Induced Liver Injury in Mice. BioMed Research International. 2017.

17. Hye Jung Park, Min Kwang Byun, Hyung Jung Kim, et al. Dietary vitamin C intake protects against COPD: the Korea National Health and Nutrition Examination Survey in 2012. International Journal of Chronic Obstructive Pulmonary Disease. 2016.

18. Yoshiko Fukuchi, Masanori Hiramitsu, Miki Okada, et al. Lemon Polyphenols Suppress Diet-induced Obesity by Up-Regulation of mRNA Levels of the Enzymes Involved in β-Oxidation in Mouse White Adipose Tissue. Journal of Clinical Biochemistry and Nutrition. 2008.

19. Migiwa Komiya, Takashi Takeuchi, Etsumori Harada. Lemon oil vapor causes an anti-stress effect via modulating the 5-HT and DA activities in mice. Behavioural Brain Research. 2006.

Tip 37 - Tea Break

1. Xiangbing Mao, Changsong Gu, Daiwen Chen, Bing Yu, and Jun He. Oxidative stress-induced diseases and tea polyphenols. Oncotarget. 2017.

2. Xinyan Wang, Fangchao Liu, Jianxin Li, et al. Tea consumption and the risk of atherosclerotic cardiovascular disease and all-cause mortality: The China-PAR project. European Journal of Preventive Cardiology. 2020.

3. Junhua Li, Rafael Romero-Garcia, John Suckling, and Lei Feng. Habitual tea drinking modulates brain efficiency: evidence from brain connectivity evaluation. Aging. 2019.

4. Edele Mancini, Christoph Beglinger, Jürgen Drewe, et al. Green tea effects on cognition, mood and human brain function: A systematic review. Phytomedicine. 2017.

5. He-Ying Hu, Bang-Sheng Wu, Ya-Nan Ou, et al. Tea consumption and risk of incident dementia: A prospective cohort study of 377 592 UK Biobank participants. Nature Translational Psychiatry. 2022.

6. Suk-Joon Hyung, Alaina S. DeToma, Jeffrey R. Brender, et al. Insights into antiamyloidogenic properties of the green tea extract

(−)-epigallocatechin-3-gallate toward metal-associated amyloid-β species. PNAS. 2013.

7. Paul M. Seidler, Kevin A. Murray, David R. Boyer, et al. Structure-based discovery of small molecules that disaggregate Alzheimer's disease tissue derived tau fibrils in vitro. Nature Communications. 2022.

8. Yanyan Wang, Maoquan Li, Xueqing Xu, et al. Green tea epigallocatechin-3-gallate (EGCG) promotes neural progenitor cell proliferation and sonic hedgehog pathway activation during adult hippocampal neurogenesis. Molecular Nutrition & Food Research. 2012.

9. Mauro Serafini, Daniele Del Rio, Denis N'Dri Yao, Saverio Bettuzzi, and Ilaria Peluso. Chapter 12 - Health Benefits of Tea. Herbal Medicine: Biomolecular and Clinical Aspects. 2nd edition. 2011.

10. Naghma Khan and Hasan Mukhtar. Tea and Health: Studies in Human. Current Pharmaceutical Design. 2013.

11. Danielle Glick, Sandra Barth, and Kay F. Macleod. Autophagy: cellular and molecular mechanisms. The Journal of Pathology. 2010.

12. Mani Iyer Prasanth, Bhagavathi Sundaram Sivamaruthi, Chaiyavat Chaiyasut, Tewin Tencomnao. A Review of the Role of Green Tea (Camellia sinensis) in Antiphotoaging, Stress Resistance, Neuroprotection, and Autophagy. Nutrients MDPI. 2019.

13. Tamsyn SA Thring, Pauline Hili & Declan P Naughton. Anti-collagenase, anti-elastase and anti-oxidant activities of extracts from 21 plants. BMC Complementary Medicine and Therapies. 2009.

14. Kyung Ok Lee, Sang Nam Kim, and Young Chul Kim. Anti-wrinkle Effects of Water Extracts of Teas in Hairless Mouse. Toxicological Research. 2014.

15. Swapna Upadhyay and Madhulika Dixit. Role of Polyphenols and Other Phytochemicals on Molecular Signaling. Oxidative Medicine and Cellular Longevity. 2015.

16. Arpita Basu, Nancy M. Betts, Afework Mulugeta, et al. Green tea supplementation increases glutathione and plasma antioxidant capacity in adults with the metabolic syndrome. Nutrition Research. 2013.

17. Kanti Bhooshan Pandey and Syed Ibrahim Rizv. Plant polyphenols as dietary antioxidants in human health and disease. Oxidative Medicine and Cellular Longevity. 2009.

18. Zafar Rasheed. Molecular evidences of health benefits of drinking black tea. International Journal of Health Sciences. 2019.
19. Brahma N. Singh, Sharmila Shankar, and Rakesh K. Srivastava. Green tea catechin, epigallocatechin-3-gallate (EGCG): mechanisms, perspectives and clinical applications. Biochemical Pharmacology. 2011.
20. Jerzy Jankun, Steven H. Selman, Rafal Swiercz & Ewa Skrzypczak-Jankun. Why drinking green tea could prevent cancer. Nature. 1997.
21. Jing Zhao, Alan Blayney, Xiaorong Liu, et al. EGCG binds intrinsically disordered N-terminal domain of p53 and disrupts p53-MDM2 interaction. Nature Communications. 2021.
22. Iman A. Hakim, Robin B. Harris, Sylvia Brown, et al. Effect of Increased Tea Consumption on Oxidative DNA Damage among Smokers. The Journal of Nutrition. 2003.
23. Bauer E Sumpio, Alfredo C Cordova, David W Berke-Schlessel, Feng Qin, Quan Hai Chen. Green Tea, the "Asian Paradox," and Cardiovascular Disease. Journal of the American College of Surgeons. 2006.
24. Gavin E Arteel, Takehiko Uesugi, Leslie N Bevan, et al. Green tea extract protects against early alcohol-induced liver injury in rats. Biological Chemistry. 2002.
25. Ryuichiro Sakata, Toru Nakamura, Takuji Torimura, Takato Ueno Michio Sata. Green tea with high-density catechins improves liver function and fat infiltration in non-alcoholic fatty liver disease (NAFLD) patients: A double-blind placebo-controlled study. International Journal of Molecular Medicine. 2013.
26. Chwan-Li Shen, James K. Yeh, Jay Cao, and Jia-Sheng Wang. Green Tea and Bone metabolism. Nutrition Research. 2009.
27. Haneen A. Abusharkh, Olivia M. Reynolds, Juana Mendenhall, et al. Combining stretching and gallic acid to decrease inflammation indices and promote extracellular matrix production in osteoarthritic human articular chondrocytes. Experimental Cell Research. 2021.
28. Tongtong Guo, Dan Song, Lu Cheng, and Xin Zhang. Interactions of tea catechins with intestinal microbiota and their implication for human health. Food Science and Biotechnology. 2019.
29. Tarun Vyas, Ravleen Nagi, Archana Bhatia, and Sandeep Kumar Bains, et al. Therapeutic effects of green tea as an antioxidant on oral health- A review. Journal of Family Medicine and Primary Care. 2021.

30. Babitha Nugala, Ambalavanan Namasi, Pamela Emmadi, and P. Mohana Krishna. Role of green tea as an antioxidant in periodontal disease: The Asian paradox. Journal of Indian Society of Periodontology. 2012.
31. Pradeep J Nathan, Kristy Lu, M Gray, C Oliver. The neuropharmacology of L-theanine(N-ethyl-L-glutamine): a possible neuroprotective and cognitive enhancing agent. Journal of Herbal Pharmacotherapy. 2006.
32. Nicole M Delimont, Mark D Haub, and Brian L Lindshield. The Impact of Tannin Consumption on Iron Bioavailability and Status: A Narrative Review. Current Developments in Nutrition. 2017.
33. A M Abd El-Aty, Jeong-Heui Choi, Md Musfiqur Rahman, et al. Residues and contaminants in tea and tea infusions: a review. Food Additives & Contaminants. 2014.

Tip 38 - Coffee's Wake Up Concerns

1. Steven E. Meredith, Laura M. Juliano, John R. Hughes, and Roland R. Griffiths. Caffeine Use Disorder: A Comprehensive Review and Research Agenda. Journal of Caffeine Research. 2013.
2. Ningjian Liang and David D. Kitts. Role of Chlorogenic Acids in Controlling Oxidative and Inflammatory Stress Conditions. Nutrients MDPI. 2016.
3. Margreet R Olthof, Peter C Hollman, Peter L Zock, Martijn B Katan. Consumption of high doses of chlorogenic acid, present in coffee, or of black tea increases plasma total homocysteine concentrations in humans. The American Journal of Clinical Nutrition. 2001.
4. Martha Sibrian-Vazquez, Jorge O. Escobedo, Soojin Lim, George K. Samoei, and Robert M. Strongin. Homocystamides promote free-radical and oxidative damage to proteins. PNAS. 2009.
5. Niloofar Kahkeshani, Soodabeh Saeidnia, and Mohammad Abdollahi. Role of antioxidants and phytochemicals on acrylamide mitigation from food and reducing its toxicity. Journal of Food Science and Technology. 2014.
6. M L Nurminen, L Niittynen, R Korpela & H Vapaatalo. Coffee, caffeine and blood pressure: a critical review. European Journal of Clinical Nutrition. 1999.
7. Antonis Zampelas, Demosthenes B Panagiotakos, Christos Pit-

savos, Christina Chrysohoou, Christodoulos Stefanadis. Associations between coffee consumption and inflammatory markers in healthy persons: the ATTICA study. The American Journal of Clinical Nutrition. 2004.

8. Sabine M. Post, Elly C. M. de Wit, and Hans M. G. Princen. Cafestol, the cholesterol-raising factor in boiled coffee, suppresses bile acid synthesis by downregulation of cholesterol 7 alpha-hydroxylase and sterol 27-hydroxylase in rat hepatocytes. Arteriosclerosis, Thrombosis, and Vascular Biology. 1997.

9. Acrylamide and Cancer Risk. National Cancer Institute. 2017.

10. Åsne Lirhus Svatun, Maja-Lisa Løchen, Dag Steinar Thelle, and Tom Wilsgaard. Association between espresso coffee and serum total cholesterol: the Tromsø Study 2015–2016. openheart. 2022.

11. Anna Gavrieli, Mary Yannakoulia, Elizabeth Fragopoulou, et al. Caffeinated Coffee Does Not Acutely Affect Energy Intake, Appetite, or Inflammation but Prevents Serum Cortisol Concentrations from Falling in Healthy Men. The Journal of Nutrition. 2011.

12. James D Lane, Carl F Pieper, Barbara G Phillips-Bute, John E Bryant, Cynthia M Kuhn. Caffeine affects cardiovascular and neuroendocrine activation at work and home. Psychosomatic Medicine. 2002.

13. Arve Ulvik, Stein Emil Vollset, Geir Hoff, Per Magne Ueland. Coffee Consumption and Circulating B-Vitamins in Healthy Middle-Aged Men and Women. Clinical Chemistry. 2008.

14. Hee-Sook Lim, Hae-Hyeog Lee, Dong-Won Byun, et al. Serum Vitamin D Level Related to Coffee Consumption in Korean Young Adults Using the 5th Korea National Health and Nutrition Examination Survey. Journal of Bone Metabolism. 2017.

15. E A Bergman, L K Massey, K J Wise, D J Sherrard. Effects of dietary caffeine on renal handling of minerals in adult women. Life Sciences. 1990.

16. Yutaka Tajima. Coffee-induced Hypokalaemia. Clinical Medicine Insights: Case Reports. 2010.

17. P S Aldrian, C L Keen, B Lönnerdal, K G Dewey. Effects of coffee consumption on iron, zinc and copper status in nonpregnant and pregnant Sprague-Dawley rats. International Journal of Food Sciences and Nutrition. 1997.

18. Harry A Smith, Aaron Hengist, Joel Thomas, et al. Glucose control upon waking is unaffected by hourly sleep fragmentation during the night, but is impaired by morning caffeinated coffee. British Journal of Nutrition. 2020.

Tip 39 - Melatonin Nightcap

1. Alina Masters, Seithikurippu R Pandi-Perumal, Azizi Seixas, Jean-Louis Girardin, and Samy I. McFarlane. Melatonin, the Hormone of Darkness: From Sleep Promotion to Ebola Treatment. Brain Disorders & Therapy. 2015.

2. Sujana Reddy; Vamsi Reddy; Sandeep Sharma. Physiology, Circadian Rhythm. StatPearls. 2021.

3. Anna Aulinas, MD, PhD. Physiology of the Pineal Gland and Melatonin. Endotext. 2000.

4. Katri Peuhkuri, Nora Sihvola, and Riitta Korpela. Dietary factors and fluctuating levels of melatonin. Food & Nutrition Research. 2012.

5. Alan G Wade, Gordon Crawford, Ian Ford, et al. Prolonged release melatonin in the treatment of primary insomnia: evaluation of the age cut-off for short- and long-term response. Current Medical Research and Opinion. 2010.

6. Elizabeth A. Thomson. Rest easy: MIT study confirms melatonin's value as sleep aid. Massachusetts Institute of Technology. 2005.

7. Annia Galano, Dun Xian Tan, Russel J Reiter. Melatonin as a natural ally against oxidative stress: a physicochemical examination. Journal of Pineal Research. 2011.

8. Ran Liu, Alan Fu, Aaron E Hoffman, Tongzhang Zheng, Yong Zhu. Melatonin enhances DNA repair capacity possibly by affecting genes involved in DNA damage responsive pathways. BMC Molecular and Cell Biology. 2013.

9. P Lissoni, S Barni, A Ardizzoia, et al. Cancer immunotherapy with low-dose interleukin-2 subcutaneous administration: potential efficacy in most solid tumor histotypes by a concomitant treatment with the pineal hormone melatonin. The Journal of Biological Regulators & Homeostatic Agents. 1993.

10. Talita da Silva Mendes de Farias, Maysa Mariana Cruz, Roberta Cavalcante da Cunha de Sa, et al. Melatonin Supplementation Decreases Hypertrophic Obesity and Inflammation Induced by High-Fat Diet in Mice. Frontiers in Endocrinology. 2019.

11. Sylvie Tordjman, Sylvie Chokron, Richard Delorme, et al. Melatonin: Pharmacology, Functions and Therapeutic Benefits. Current Neuropharmacology. 2017.

12. Ifigenia Kostoglou-Athanassiou. Therapeutic applications of melatonin. Endocrinology and Metabolism. 2013.

13. A J Billyard, D L Eggett, K B Franz. Dietary magnesium deficiency decreases plasma melatonin in rats. Magnesium Research. 2006.
14. Lauren A.E. Erland, MSc, Praveen K. Saxena, PhD. Melatonin Natural Health Products and Supplements: Presence of Serotonin and Significant Variability of Melatonin Content. Journal of Clinical Sleep Medicine. 2017.
15. Haruna Fukushige, Yumi Fukuda, Mizuho Tanaka, et al. Effects of tryptophan-rich breakfast and light exposure during the daytime on melatonin secretion at night. Journal of Physiological Anthropology. 2014.

Tip 40 - Your Tongue is a Window Into Your Health

1. Maureen Stone, Jonghye Woo, Junghoon Lee, et al. Structure and variability in human tongue muscle anatomy. Computer Methods in Biomechanics and Biomedical Engineering. 2016.
2. Bruno Bordoni, Bruno Morabito, Roberto Mitrano, Marta Simonelli, and Anastasia Toccafondi. The Anatomical Relationships of the Tongue with the Body System. Cureus. 2018.
3. Martin Edwards. Put Out Your Tongue! The Role of Clinical Insight in the Study of the History of Medicine. International Journal for the History of Medicine and Related Sciences. 2011.
4. Tsung-Chieh Lee, Lun-Chien Lo, and Fang-Chen Wu. Traditional Chinese Medicine for Metabolic Syndrome via TCM Pattern Differentiation: Tongue Diagnosis for Predictor. Evidence-Based Complementary and Alternative Medicine. 2016.
5. Mingfeng Zhu, Jianqiang Du, and Chenghua Ding. A Comparative Study of Contemporary Color Tongue Image Extraction Methods Based on HSI. Evidence-Based Complementary and Alternative Medicine. 2014.

Tip 41 - Beating Gout

1. George Nuki & Peter A Simkin. A concise history of gout and hyperuricemia and their treatment. Arthritis Research & Therapy. 2006.
2. Pooja Poudel; Amandeep Goyal; Pankaj Bansal; Sarah L. Lappin. Inflammatory Arthritis. StatPearls. 2021.
3. Eswar Krishnan. Hyperuricemia and Incident Heart Failure.

Circulation: Heart Failure. 2009.

4. Augustin Latourte, Aicha Soumaré, Thomas Bardin, Fernando Perez-Ruiz, Stéphanie Debette, Pascal Richette. Uric acid and incident dementia over 12 years of follow-up: a population-based cohort study. Annals of the Rheumatic Diseases. 2017.

5. Christina George; David A. Minter. Hyperuricemia. StatPearls. 2021.

6. Miguel A. Martillo, Lama Nazzal, and Daria B. Crittenden. The Crystallization of Monosodium Urate. Current Rheumatology Reports. 2014.

7. Walter G. Barr. Clinical Methods: The History, Physical, and Laboratory Examinations. 3rd edition. Chapter 165 Uric Acid. 1990.

8. Hyon K. Choi, Gary Curhan. Beer, liquor, and wine consumption and serum uric acid level: the Third National Health and Nutrition Examination Survey. Arthritis & Rheumatism. 2004.

9. S Ebrahimpour-Koujan, P Saneei, B Larijani, A Esmaillzadeh. Consumption of sugar-sweetened beverages and serum uric acid concentrations: a systematic review and meta-analysis. Journal of Human Nutrition and Dietetics. 2020.

10. Hyon K. Choi, MD, DrPH; Xiang Gao, MD, PhD; Gary Curhan, MD, ScD. Vitamin C Intake and the Risk of Gout in Men: A Prospective Study. JAMA Internal Medicine. 2009.

11. Hongjing Wang, Liping Cheng, Dingbo Lin, Zhaocheng Ma, Xiuxin Deng. Lemon fruits lower the blood uric acid levels in humans and mice. Scientia Horticulturae. 2017.

12. Yiying Zhang and Hongbin Qiu. Folate, Vitamin B6 and Vitamin B12 Intake in Relation to Hyperuricemia. Journal of Clinical Medicine. 2018.

13. Pei-En Chen, Chia-Yu Liu, Wu-Hsiung Chien, Ching-Wen Chien, and Tao-Hsin Tung. Effectiveness of Cherries in Reducing Uric Acid and Gout: A Systematic Review. Evidence-Based Complementary and Alternative Medicine. 2019.

14. Kyle Jablonski, Nicholas A. Young, Caitlin Henry, et al. Physical activity prevents acute inflammation in a gout model by downregulation of TLR2 on circulating neutrophils as well as inhibition of serum CXCL1 and is associated with decreased pain and inflammation in gout patients. PLOS ONE. 2020.

Tip 42 - A Daily Parasite Protection Plan

1. F. E. G. Cox. History of Human Parasitology. Clinical Microbiology Reviews. 2002.

2. Charlotte E Egan, Sara B Cohen, and Eric Y Denkers. Insights into inflammatory bowel disease using Toxoplasma gondii as an infectious trigger. Immunology & Cell Biology. 2011.

3. Elizabeth M. Hechenbleikner, MD and Jennifer A. McQuade, MD. Parasitic Colitis. Clinics in Colon and Rectal Surgery. 2015.

4. Rasoul Mohammadi, Ahmad Hosseini-Safa, Mohammad Javad Ehsani Ardakani, and Mohammad Rostami-Nejad. The relationship between intestinal parasites and some immune-mediated intestinal conditions. Gastroenterology and Hepatology from Bed to Bench. 2015.

5. Arturo Carpio, Matthew L. Romo, R. M. E. Parkhouse, et al. Parasitic diseases of the central nervous system: lessons for clinicians and policy makers. Expert Review of Neurotherapeutics. 2016.

6. Doodipala Samba Reddy, Randy Volkmer II. Neurocysticercosis as an infectious acquired epilepsy worldwide. Seizure. 2017.

7. Matthew Prior. Can you 'catch' cancer? Frontiers Science News. 2019.

8. James M. Hodge, Anna E. Coghill, Youngchul Kim, et al. Toxoplasma gondii infection and the risk of adult glioma in two prospective studies. International Journal of Cancer. 2021.

9. Margarida Azevedo, MSc. Research Points to Neurodegenerative Consequences, Such as ALS, of Toxoplasma Gondii Infection. ALS News Today. 2016.

10. Clément N David, Elma S Frias, Jenny I Szu, et al. GLT-1-Dependent Disruption of CNS Glutamate Homeostasis and Neuronal Function by the Protozoan Parasite Toxoplasma gondii. PLOS PATHOGENS. 2016.

11. Samantha J. Batista, Katherine M. Still, David Johanson, et al. Gasdermin-D-dependent IL-1α release from microglia promotes protective immunity during chronic Toxoplasma gondii infection. Nature Communications. 2020.

12. Y. Zhou and N. C. Danbolt. Glutamate as a neurotransmitter in the healthy brain. Journal of Neural Transmission. 2014.

13. Rashidul Haque. Human Intestinal Parasites. Journal of Health, Population and Nutrition. 2007.

14. Soil-transmitted helminth infections. World Health Organization (WHO). 2020.

15. Richard Cummings and Salvatore Turco. Chapter 40 - Parasitic

Infections. Essentials of Glycobiology. 2015.
16. Elizabeth M. Hechenbleikner, MD and Jennifer A. McQuade, MD. Parasitic Colitis. Thieme Clinics in Colon and Rectal Surgery. 2015.
17. Meagan A. Rubel, Arwa Abbas, Louis J. Taylor, et al. Lifestyle and the presence of helminths is associated with gut microbiome composition in Cameroonians. Genome Biology. 2020.
18. Darshna Yagnik, Vlad Serafin, and Ajit J. Shah. Antimicrobial activity of apple cider vinegar against Escherichia coli, Staphylococcus aureus and Candida albicans; downregulating cytokine and microbial protein expression. Scientific Reports. 2018.
19. Darshna Yagnik, Malcolm Ward, and Ajit J. Shah. Antibacterial apple cider vinegar eradicates methicillin resistant Staphylococcus aureus and resistant Escherichia coli. Scientific Reports. 2021.
20. Sultan F Alnomasy. In vitro and in vivo Anti-Toxoplasma Effects of Allium sativum Essential Oil Against Toxoplasma gondii RH Strain. Dovepress Infection and Drug Resistance. 2021.
21. Mark Force, William S. Sparks, Robert A. Ronzio. Inhibition of enteric parasites by emulsified oil of oregano in vivo. Phytotherapy Research. 2000.
22. Daniela de Paula Aguiar, Mayara Brunetto Moreira Moscardini, Enyara Rezende Morais, et al. Curcumin Generates Oxidative Stress and Induces Apoptosis in Adult Schistosoma mansoni Worms. PLOS ONE. 2016.
23. Diego Francisco Cortés-Rojas, Claudia Regina Fernandes de Souza, and Wanderley Pereira Oliveira. Clove (Syzygium aromaticum): a precious spice. Asian Pacific Journal of Tropical Biomedicine. 2014.
24. Marcelo Hisano, Homero Bruschini, Antonio Carlos Nicodemo, and Miguel Srougi. Cranberries and lower urinary tract infection prevention. Clinics. 2012.
25. Kurt Z. Long, Jorge L. Rosado, Yura Montoya, et al. Effect of vitamin A and zinc supplementation on gastrointestinal parasitic infections among Mexican children. Pediatrics. 2007.
26. John P. Heggers, John Cottingham, Jean Gusman, et al. The Effectiveness of Processed Grapefruit-Seed Extract as An Antibacterial Agent: II. Mechanism of Action and In Vitro Toxicity. The Journal of Alternative and Complementary Medicine. 2004.
27. Khanh-Van Ho, Zhentian Lei, Lloyd W. Sumner, et al. Identifying Antibacterial Compounds in Black Walnuts (Juglans nigra)

Using a Metabolomics Approach. Metabolites MDPI. 2018.

28. Xiaoyu Shi, Meng Wei, Zihao Xu, et al. Vitamin C Inhibits Blood-Stage Plasmodium Parasites via Oxidative Stress. Frontiers in Cell and Developmental Biology. 2021.

29. Marilyn F. Scott, Kristine G. Koski. Zinc Deficiency Impairs Immune Responses against Parasitic Nematode Infections at Intestinal and Systemic Sites. The Journal of Nutrition. 2000.

Tip 43 - Controlling Stress

1. David S. Goldstein. Adrenal Responses to Stress. Cellular and Molecular Neurobiology. 2010.

2. Justin B. Echouffo-Tcheugui, Sarah C. Conner, Jayandra J Himali, et al. Circulating cortisol and cognitive and structural brain measures. Neurology. 2018.

3. Eun Joo Kim, Blake Pellman, and Jeansok J. Kim. Stress effects on the hippocampus: a critical review. Learning & Memory. 2015.

4. Natalie L. Marchant, Lise R. Lovland, Rebecca Jones, et al. Repetitive negative thinking is associated with amyloid, tau, and cognitive decline. Alzheimer's & Dementia. 2020.

5. George S Bloom, PhD. Amyloid-β and tau: the trigger and bullet in Alzheimer disease pathogenesis. JAMA Neurology. 2014.

6. Earl Nightingale. Wikipedia. 2022.

7. Earl Nightingale. The Miracle of Your Mind. Premier Business Global Consultants. YouTube. 2014.

8. Habib Yaribeygi, Yunes Panahi, Hedayat Sahraei, Thomas P. Johnston, and Amirhossein Sahebkar. The impact of stress on body function: A review. EXCLI Journal. 2017.

9. Eric T Klopack, Eileen M Crimmins, Steve W Cole, et al. Social stressors associated with age-related T lymphocyte percentages in older US adults: Evidence from the US Health and Retirement Study. PNAS. 2022.

10. Melanie D Hingle, Betsy C Wertheim, Hilary A Tindle, et al. Optimism and diet quality in the Women's Health Initiative. Journal of the Academy of Nutrition and Dietetics. 2013.

11. Ciro Conversano, Alessandro Rotondo, Elena Lensi, et al. Optimism and Its Impact on Mental and Physical Well-Being. Clinical Practice & Epidemiology in Mental Health. 2010.

12. Ai Ikeda, Joel Schwartz, Junenette L Peters, et al. Optimism in Relation to Inflammation and Endothelial Dysfunction in Older Men: The VA Normative Aging Study. Psychosomatic Medicine. 2011.
13. Alan Rozanski, Chirag Bavishi, Laura D Kubzansky, et al. Association of Optimism With Cardiovascular Events and All-Cause Mortality. JAMA Network Open. 2019.
14. Adrian L Lopresti. The Effects of Psychological and Environmental Stress on Micronutrient Concentrations in the Body: A Review of the Evidence. Advances in Nutrition. 2020.

Tip 44 - Preventing and Reversing Gray Hairs

1. Ayelet M Rosenberg, Shannon Rausser, Junting Ren, et al. Quantitative mapping of human hair greying and reversal in relation to life stress. eLife. 2021.
2. Djahida Bedja, Wenwen Yan, Viren Lad, et al. Inhibition of glycosphingolipid synthesis reverses skin inflammation and hair loss in ApoE−/− mice fed western diet. Scientific Reports. 2018.
3. Ralph M Trüeb. Oxidative Stress in Ageing of Hair. International Journal of Trichology. 2009.
4. Deepashree Daulatabad, Archana Singal, Chander Grover, et al. Assessment of Oxidative Stress in Patients with Premature Canities. International Journal of Trichology. 2015.
5. Seong Kyeong Jo, Ji Yeon Lee, Young Lee, Chang Deok Kim, Jeung-Hoon Lee, and Young Ho Lee. Three Streams for the Mechanism of Hair Graying. Annals of Dermatology. 2018.
6. Mirosława Cichorek, Małgorzata Wachulska, Aneta Stasiewicz, and Agata Tymińska. Skin melanocytes: biology and development. Advances in Dermatology and Allergology. 2013.
7. Bing Zhang, Sai Ma, Inbal Rachmin, et al. Hyperactivation of sympathetic nerves drives depletion of melanocyte stem cells. Nature. 2020.
8. Andreas M Finner, MD. Nutrition and hair: deficiencies and supplements. Dermatologic Clinics. 2013.
9. Male-pattern baldness and premature greying associated with risk of early heart disease. European Society of Cardiology. 2017.
10. Fei-Chi Yang, Yuchen Zhang, and Maikel C. Rheinstädter. The structure of people's hair. PeerJ. 2014.

11. Christine A. VanBuren and Helen B. Everts. Vitamin A in Skin and Hair: An Update. Nutrients MDPI. 2022.
12. Berislav Momčilović, Ninoslav Mimica, and Juraj Prejac. Entanglement of Hair Iodine and Selenium Nutritional Status. Current Developments in Nutrition. 2020.
13. Zuzanna Rzepka, Ewa Buszman, Artur Beberok, Dorota Wrześniok. From tyrosine to melanin: Signaling pathways and factors regulating melanogenesis. Advances in Hygiene and Experimental Medicine. 2016.
14. Aaron Bunsen Lerner and Thomas B. Fitzpatrick. BIOCHEMISTRY OF MELANIN FORMATION. Department of Dermatology and Syphilology, University of Michigan. 1950.
15. Min Seong Kil, Chul Woo Kim, and Sang Seok Kim. Analysis of Serum Zinc and Copper Concentrations in Hair Loss. Annals of Dermatology. 2013.
16. A.F. Hamel, M.T. Menard, and M.A. Novak. Fatty Acid supplements improve hair coat condition in rhesus macaques. Journal of Medical Primatology. 2018.
17. Nina van Beek, Enikő Bodó, Arno Kromminga, et al. Thyroid Hormones Directly Alter Human Hair Follicle Functions: Anagen Prolongation and Stimulation of Both Hair Matrix Keratinocyte Proliferation and Hair Pigmentation. The Journal of Clinical Endocrinology & Metabolism. 2008.
18. Alshimaa M El-Sheikh, Nashwa N Elfar, Heba A Mourad, and El-Sayed S Hewedy. Relationship between Trace Elements and Premature Hair Graying. International Journal of Trichology. 2018.
19. Chris J.D. Zarafonetis, MD. Darkening of gray hair during para-amino-benzoic acid therapy. University of Michigan School of Medicine. 1950.
20. Ying Shi, Long-Fei Luo, Xiao-Ming Liu, et al. Premature Graying as a Consequence of Compromised Antioxidant Activity in Hair Bulb Melanocytes and Their Precursors. PLOS ONE. 2014.

Tip 45 - Resistance (Isometric) Exercises: A 20 Minute Workout and Detox Routine

1. Miguel J. Rodriguez. Therapeutic Exercise in General Practice. Western Journal of Medicine. 1961.
2. Laura V. Schaefer and Frank N. Bittmann. Are there two forms

of isometric muscle action? Results of the experimental study support a distinction between a holding and a pushing isometric muscle function. BMC Sports Science, Medicine and Rehabilitation. 2017.

3. Danny Lum, Tiago M Barbosa. Brief Review: Effects of Isometric Strength Training on Strength and Dynamic Performance. International Journal of Sports Medicine. 2019.

4. Priscilla M. Clarkson, Walter Kroll & Thomas C. McBride. Maximal isometric strength and fiber type composition in power and endurance athletes. European Journal of Applied Physiology and Occupational Physiology. 1980.

5. Kaleen M. Lavin, Brandon M. Roberts, Christopher S. Fry, et al. The Importance of Resistance Exercise Training to Combat Neuromuscular Aging. American Physiology Society. 2019.

6. Dustin J Oranchuk, Adam G Storey, André R Nelson, John B Cronin. Isometric training and long-term adaptations: Effects of muscle length, intensity, and intent: A systematic review. Scandinavian Journal of Medicine & Science in Sports. 2019.

7. Hyun-Seung Rhyu, Hun-Kyung Park, Jung-Sub Park, Hye-Sang Park. The effects of isometric exercise types on pain and muscle activity in patients with low back pain. Journal of Exercise Rehabilitation. 2015.

8. A Ram Hong and Sang Wan Kim. Effects of Resistance Exercise on Bone Health. Endocrinology and Metabolism. 2018.

9. Shahnawaz Anwer, MPT and Ahmad Alghadir, MS, PhD, PT. Effect of Isometric Quadriceps Exercise on Muscle Strength, Pain, and Function in Patients with Knee Osteoarthritis: A Randomized Controlled Study. Journal of Physical Therapy Science. 2014.

10. Kyle Mandsager, Serge Harb, Paul Cremer, et al. Association of Cardiorespiratory Fitness With Long-term Mortality Among Adults Undergoing Exercise Treadmill Testing. JAMA Network Open. 2018.

11. RJ Korthuis. Chapter 2 - Anatomy of Skeletal Muscle and Its Vascular Supply. Skeletal Muscle Circulation. 2011.

12. G A Rongen, J P van Dijk, E E van Ginneken, et al. Repeated ischaemic isometric exercise increases muscle fibre conduction velocity in humans: involvement of Na^+-K^+-ATPase. The Journal of Physiology. 2002.

13. Debra J Carlson, Gudrun Dieberg, Nicole C Hess, Philip J Millar, Neil A Smart. Isometric exercise training for blood pressure management: a systematic review and meta-analysis. Mayo. 2014.

Tip 46 - Why We Need Sunshine (Vitamin D)

1. Stephen J. Genuis, MD. Keeping your sunny side up: How sunlight affects health and well-being. Canadian Family Physician Journal. 2006.
2. Robert Briggs, Kevin McCarroll, Aisling O'Halloran, et al. Vitamin D Deficiency Is Associated With an Increased Likelihood of Incident Depression in Community-Dwelling Older Adults. JAMDA. 2019.
3. Rathish Nair and Arun Maseeh. Vitamin D: The "sunshine" vitamin. Journal of Pharmacology & Pharmacotherapeutics. 2012.
4. Michael F. Holick, Ph.D., M.D. Vitamin D Status: Measurement, Interpretation, and Clinical Application. Annals of Epidemiology. 2009.
5. Meenakshi Umar, Konduru S. Sastry, and Aouatef I. Chouchane. Role of Vitamin D Beyond the Skeletal Function: A Review of the Molecular and Clinical Studies. International Journal of Molecule Sciences. 2018.
6. What is Osteoporosis and What Causes It? National Osteoporosis Foundation. 2022.
7. Hanmin Wang, Weiwen Chen, Dongqing Li, et al. Vitamin D and Chronic Diseases. Aging and Disease. 2017.
8. Jonghoo Lee, Hye Kyeong Park, Min-Jung Kwon, et al. Decreased lung function is associated with vitamin D deficiency in apparently health, middle aged Koreans: the Kangbuk Samsung Health Study. European Journal of Clinical Nutrition. 2020.
9. Cedric F. Garland, DrPH, Frank C. Garland, PhD, Edward D. Gorham, PhD, MPH, et al. The Role of Vitamin D in Cancer Prevention. AJPH. 2006.
10. F C Garland, M R White, C F Garland, E Shaw, E D Gorham. Occupational sunlight exposure and melanoma in the U.S. Navy. Archives of Environmental Health: An International Journal. 1990.
11. Dr. Zahid Naeem. Vitamin D Deficiency- An Ignored Epidemic. 2010. International Journal of Health Sciences. 2010.
12. David G. Hoel, Marianne Berwick, Frank R. de Gruijl, and Michael F. Holick. The risks and benefits of sun exposure 2016. Dermato-Endocrinology. 2016.
13. Alexander Michels, PhD. Can You Rely on Sunlight to Get Enough Vitamin D This Winter? Linus Pauling Institute. 2016.

14. Vitamin D. National Institutes of Health, Office of Dietary Supplements. 2021.

15. Michael F. Holick, Neil C. Binkley, Heike A. Bischoff-Ferrari, et al. Evaluation, Treatment, and Prevention of Vitamin D Deficiency: an Endocrine Society Clinical Practice Guideline. The Journal of Clinical Endocrinology & Metabolism. 2011.

16. Qi Dai, Xiangzhu Zhu, JoAnn E Manson, et al. Magnesium status and supplementation influence vitamin D status and metabolism: results from a randomized trial. The American Journal of Clinical Nutrition. 2018.

17. Lisa A Houghton, Reinhold Vieth. The case against ergocalciferol (vitamin D2) as a vitamin supplement. The American Journal of Clinical Nutrition. 2006.

18. Laura Tripkovic, Helen Lambert, Kathryn Hart, et al. Comparison of vitamin D2 and vitamin D3 supplementation in raising serum 25-hydroxyvitamin D status: a systematic review and meta-analysis. The American Journal of Clinical Nutrition. 2012.

19. Victoria F Logan, Andrew R Gray, Meredith C Peddie, Michelle J Harper, Lisa A Houghton. Long-term vitamin D3 supplementation is more effective than vitamin D2 in maintaining serum 25-hydroxyvitamin D status over the winter months. British Journal of Nutrition. 2012.

20. Joshua M. Schulman and David E. Fisher. Indoor UV tanning and skin cancer: health risks and opportunities. Current Opinion in Oncology. 2009.

21. Sunbeds and UV Radiation. International Agency for Research on Cancer (IARC). 2009.

22. Kim M. Pfotenhauer and Jay H. Shubrook. Vitamin D Deficiency, Its Role in Health and Disease, and Current Supplementation Recommendations. Journal of American Osteopathic Association. 2017.

23. The Trouble With Ingredients in Sunscreens. Environmental Working Group. 2020.

24. Gillian L Fell, Kathleen C Robinson, Jianren Mao, et al. Skin β-endorphin mediates addiction to UV light. Cell. 2014.

25. G W Lambert, C Reid, D M Kaye, G L Jennings, M D Esler. Effect of sunlight and season on serotonin turnover in the brain. The Lancet. 2002.

26. Simon N. Young. How to increase serotonin in the human brain without drugs. Journal of Psychiatry & Neuroscience. 2007.

Tip 47 - Brewer's Yeast: A Complete Meal

1. Hiren Karathia, Ester Vilaprinyo, Albert Sorribas, and Rui Alves. Saccharomyces cerevisiae as a Model Organism: A Comparative Study. PLOS ONE. 2011.

2. Mark A Moyad. Brewer's/baker's yeast (Saccharomyces cerevisiae) and preventive medicine: part I. Urologic Nurses. 2007

3. Isabel X. Wang, Christopher Grunseich, Youree G. Chung, et al. RNA–DNA sequence differences in Saccharomyces cerevisiae. Genome Research. 2016.

4. Tahereh Tahmasebi, Rahim Nosrati, Hamed Zare, et al. Isolation of indigenous Glutathione producing Saccharomyces cerevisiae strains. IJP. 2016.

5. Kate Petersen Shay, Régis F. Moreau, Eric J. Smith, Anthony R. Smith, and Tory M. Hagen. Alpha-lipoic acid as a dietary supplement: Molecular mechanisms and therapeutic potential. Biochimica et Biophysica Acta (BBA) - General Subjects. 2009.

6. Suat Kucukgoncu, Elton Zhou, Katherine B Lucas, and Cenk Tek. Alpha-Lipoic Acid (ALA) as a supplementation for weight loss: Results from a Meta-Analysis of Randomized Controlled Trials. Obesity Reviews. 2017.

7. Agape M. Awad, Michelle C. Bradley, Lucía Fernández-del-Río, et al. Coenzyme Q10 deficiencies: pathways in yeast and humans. Essays in Biochemistry. 2018.

8. Amino acids. National Institutes of Health (NIH). MedlinePlus. 2022.

9. Abdulla A.-B. Badawy, Donald M. Dougherty, and Dawn M. Richard. Specificity of the Acute Tryptophan and Tyrosine Plus Phenylalanine Depletion and Loading Tests I. Review of Biochemical Aspects and Poor Specificity of Current Amino Acid Formulations. International Journal of Tryptophan Research. 2010.

10. Patricia Hildebrand, Werner Königschulte, Tilman Jakob Gaber, et al. Effects of dietary tryptophan and phenylalanine–tyrosine depletion on phasic alertness in healthy adults – A pilot study. Food & Nutrition Research. 2015.

11. Takashi Takahashi, Fei Yu, Shi-jie Zhu, Junji Moriya, et al. Beneficial Effect of Brewers' Yeast Extract on Daily Activity in a Murine Model of Chronic Fatigue Syndrome. Evidence-Based Complementary and Alternative Medicine. 2006.

12. Eunice A Yamada, Valdemiro C Sgarbieri. Yeast (Saccharomyces

cerevisiae) protein concentrate: preparation, chemical composition, and nutritional and functional properties. Journal of Agricultural and Food Chemistry. 2006.

13. Heike Stier, Veronika Ebbeskotte, and Joerg Gruenwald. Immune-modulatory effects of dietary Yeast Beta-1,3/1,6-D-glucan. Nutritional Journal. 2014.

14. Annegret Auinger, Linda Riede, Gordana Bothe, et al. Yeast (1,3)-(1,6)-beta-glucan helps to maintain the body's defence against pathogens: a double-blind, randomized, placebo-controlled, multicentric study in healthy subjects. European Journal of Nutrition. 2013.

15. Mark A Moyad, Larry E Robinson, Edward T Zawada, et al. Immunogenic yeast-based fermentate for cold/flu-like symptoms in nonvaccinated individuals. The Journal of Alternative and Complementary Medicine. 2010.

16. Amir Saber, Beitollah Alipour, Zeinab Faghfoori, Ahmad Yari Khosroushahi. Cellular and molecular effects of yeast probiotics on cancer. Critical Reviews in Microbiology. 2016.

Tip 48 - Berries Are Brain Food

1. Selvaraju Subash, Musthafa Mohamed Essa, Ph.D., Samir Al-Adawi, et al. Neuroprotective effects of berry fruits on neurodegenerative diseases. Neural Regeneration Research. 2014.

2. Joanna L. Bowtell, Zainie Aboo-Bakkar, Myra E. Conway, et al. Enhanced task-related brain activation and resting perfusion in healthy older adults after chronic blueberry supplementation. Applied Physiology, Nutrition, and Metabolism. 2017.

3. Sona Skrovankova, Daniela Sumczynski, Jiri Mlcek, Tunde Jurikova, Jiri Sochor. Bioactive Compounds and Antioxidant Activity in Different Types of Berries. International Journal of Molecular Sciences. 2015.

4. Shama V. Joseph, Indika Edirisinghe, and Britt M. Burton-Freeman. Berries: anti-inflammatory effects in humans. Journal of Agricultural and Food Chemistry. 2014.

5. James A. Joseph, Barbara Shukitt-Hale, Natalia A. Denisova, et al. Reversals of Age-Related Declines in Neuronal Signal Transduction, Cognitive, and Motor Behavioral Deficits with Blueberry, Spinach, or Strawberry Dietary Supplementation. The Journal of Neuroscience. 1999.

6. Carol L. Cheatham, L. Grant Canipe III, Grace Millsap, et al. Six-month intervention with wild blueberries improved speed

of processing in mild cognitive decline: a double-blind, placebo-controlled, randomized clinical trial. Nutritional Neuroscience. 2022.

7. Sanne Ahles, Peter J. Joris, and Jogchum Plat. Effects of Berry Anthocyanins on Cognitive Performance, Vascular Function and Cardiometabolic Risk Markers: A Systematic Review of Randomized Placebo-Controlled Intervention Studies in Humans. International Journal of Molecular Sciences MDPI. 2021.

8. Julien Bensalem, PhD, Stéphanie Dudonné, PhD, Nicole Etchamendy, PhD, et al. Elderly with Lower Level of Memory Performance: A Bicentric Double-Blind, Randomized, Placebo-Controlled Clinical Study. The Journals of Gerontology. 2019.

9. Octavio Paredes-López, Martha L Cervantes-Ceja, Mónica Vigna-Pérez, Talía Hernández-Pérez. Berries: improving human health and healthy aging, and promoting quality life--a review. Plant Foods for Human Nutrition. 2010.

10. Pan Pan and Li-Shu Wang. Advancing berry research in cancer. Journal of Berry Research. 2018.

11. Haohai Huang, Guangzhao Chen, Dan Liao, Yongkun Zhu, and Xiaoyan Xue. Effects of Berries Consumption on Cardiovascular Risk Factors: A Meta-analysis with Trial Sequential Analysis of Randomized Controlled Trials. Scientific Reports. 2016.

12. Vanessa Garcia-Larsen, James F. Potts, Ernst Omenaas, et al. Dietary antioxidants and 10-year lung function decline in adults from the ECRHS survey. European Respiratory Journal. 2017

Tip 49 - Omega Fatty Acids Build and Maintain a Healthy Head

1. Anthony A. Mercadante; Prasanna Tadi. Neuroanatomy, Gray Matter. StatPearls. 2020.

2. Claudia L. Satizabal, Jayandra Jung Himali, Alexa S. Beiser, et al. Association of Red Blood Cell Omega-3 Fatty Acids With MRI Markers and Cognitive Function in Midlife: The Framingham Heart Study. Neurology. 2022.

3. Mateusz Cholewski, Monika Tomczykowa, and Michał Tomczyk. A Comprehensive Review of Chemistry, Sources and Bioavailability of Omega-3 Fatty Acids. Nutrients MDPI. 2018.

4. Daniel G Amen, William S Harris, Parris M Kidd, Somayeh Meysami, Cyrus A Raji. Quantitative Erythrocyte Omega-3 EPA Plus DHA Levels are Related to Higher Regional Cerebral Blood Flow on Brain SPECT. Journal of Alzheimer's Disease. 2017.

5. Raquel Marin. The neuronal membrane as a key factor in neurodegeneration. Frontiers in Physiology. 2013.
6. Yihui Shen, Zhilun Zhao, Luyuan Zhang, et al. Metabolic activity induces membrane phase separation in endoplasmic reticulum. PNAS. 2017.
7. Mark Hamer, G. David Batty. Association of body mass index and waist-to-hip ratio with brain structure: UK Biobank study. Neurology. 2019.
8. J. Thomas, C. J. Thomas, J. Radcliffe, and C. Itsiopoulos. Omega-3 Fatty Acids in Early Prevention of Inflammatory Neurodegenerative Disease: A Focus on Alzheimer's Disease. BioMed Research International. 2015.
9. S Kalmijn, L J Launer, A Ott, et al. Dietary fat intake and the risk of incident dementia in the Rotterdam Study. Annals of Neurology. 1997.
10. Kuan-Pin Su, Ping-Tao Tseng, Pao-Yen Lin, et al. Association of Use of Omega-3 Polyunsaturated Fatty Acids With Changes in Severity of Anxiety Symptoms. JAMA Network Open. 2018.
11. Jalal Shakeri, Maryam Khanegi, Sanobar Golshani, et al. Effects of Omega-3 Supplement in the Treatment of Patients with Bipolar I Disorder. International Journal of Preventive Medicine. 2016.
12. Jane Pei-Chen Chang, Kuan-Pin Su, Valeria Mondelli, et al. High-dose eicosapentaenoic acid (EPA) improves attention and vigilance in children and adolescents with attention deficit hyperactivity disorder (ADHD) and low endogenous EPA levels. Translational Psychiatry. 2019.
13. Joseph. R. Hibbelna and Rachel V. Gow. Omega-3 Fatty Acid and Nutrient Deficits in Adverse Neurodevelopment and Childhood Behaviors. Child and Adolescent Psychiatric Clinics of North America. 2015.
14. Gerard Hornstra. Essential fatty acids in mothers and their neonates. The American Journal of Clinical Nutrition. 2000.
15. A. Veronica Witte, Lucia Kerti, Henrike M. Hermannstädter, et al. Long-Chain Omega-3 Fatty Acids Improve Brain Function and Structure in Older Adults. Cerebral Cortex. 2014.
16. L Penke, S Muñoz Maniega, M E Bastin, et al. Brain white matter tract integrity as a neural foundation for general intelligence. Nature Molecular Psychiatry. 2012.
17. Christopher M. Filley, M.D. White Matter Dementia: Origin, Development, Progress, and Prospects. The Journal of Neuro-

psychiatry and Clinical Neurosciences. 2016.

18. Nicolas Blondeau, Robert H. Lipsky, Miled Bourourou, et al. Alpha-Linolenic Acid: An Omega-3 Fatty Acid with Neuroprotective Properties—Ready for Use in the Stroke Clinic? BioMed Research International. 2015.

19. Philip C Calder. Docosahexaenoic Acid. Annals of Nutrition and Metabolism. 2016.

20. S Yehuda, S Rabinovitz, D I Mostofsky. Essential fatty acids and the brain: from infancy to aging. Neurobiology of Aging. 2005.

21. Nir Erdinest; Or Shmueli; Yoni Grossman; Haim Ovadia; Abraham Solomon. Anti-Inflammatory Effects of Alpha Linolenic Acid on Human Corneal Epithelial Cells. Investigative Ophthalmology & Visual Science. 2012.

22. Parris M Kidd. Omega-3 DHA and EPA for cognition, behavior, and mood: clinical findings and structural-functional synergies with cell membrane phospholipids. Alternative Medicine Review. 2007.

23. Michael J. Weiser, Christopher M. Butt, and M. Hasan Mohajeri. Docosahexaenoic Acid and Cognition throughout the Lifespan. Nutrients MDPI. 2016.

24. Simon C. Dyall. Long-chain omega-3 fatty acids and the brain: a review of the independent and shared effects of EPA, DPA and DHA. Frontiers in Aging Neuroscience. 2015.

25. Fernando Gómez-Pinilla. Brain foods: the effects of nutrients on brain function. Nature Reviews Neuroscience. 2010.

26. Y Zhang, P Zhuang, W He, et al. Association of fish and long-chain omega-3 fatty acids intakes with total and cause-specific mortality: prospective analysis of 421 309 individuals. Journal of Internal Medicine. 2018.

27. William S. Harris, Nathan L. Tintle, Fumiaki Imamura, et al. Blood n-3 fatty acid levels and total and cause-specific mortality from 17 prospective studies. Nature Communications. 2021.

28. Ramin Farzaneh-Far, MD; Jue Lin, PhD; Elissa S. Epel, PhD, et al. Association of Marine Omega-3 Fatty Acid Levels With Telomeric Aging in Patients With Coronary Heart Disease. JAMA Network. 2010.

29. alpha-Linolenic acid. Wikipedia. 2022.

30. Frédéric Darios, Bazbek Davletov. Omega-3 and omega-6 fatty acids stimulate cell membrane expansion by acting on syntaxin 3. Nature. 2006.

31. Matti Marklund, Jason H Y Wu, Fumiaki Imamura, et al. Biomarkers of Dietary Omega-6 Fatty Acids and Incident Cardiovascular Disease and Mortality. Circulation. 2019.

32. E. Patterson, R. Wall, G. F. Fitzgerald, R. P. Ross, and C. Stanton. Health Implications of High Dietary Omega-6 Polyunsaturated Fatty Acids. Journal of Nutrition and Metabolism. 2012.

33. A P Simopoulos. The importance of the ratio of omega-6/omega-3 essential fatty acids. Biomedicine & Pharmacotherapy. 2002.

34. Juhee Song, Joohyeok Park, Jinyeong Jung, et al. Analysis of Trans Fat in Edible Oils with Cooking Process. Toxicological Research. 2015.

35. Zhi-Hao Li, Wen-Fang Zhong, Simin Liu, et al. Associations of habitual fish oil supplementation with cardiovascular outcomes and all cause mortality: evidence from a large population based cohort study. BMJ. 2020.

36. Ronald A Hites, Jeffery A Foran, David O Carpenter, et al. Global Assessment of Organic Contaminants in Farmed Salmon. Science. 2004.

37. David Cameron-Smith, Benjamin B. Albert, and Wayne S. Cutfield, Fishing for answers: is oxidation of fish oil supplements a problem? Journal of Nutritional Science. 2015.

38. Giuseppe Grosso, Fabio Galvano, Stefano Marventano, et al. Omega-3 Fatty Acids and Depression: Scientific Evidence and Biological Mechanisms. Oxidative Medicine and Cellular Longevity. 2014.

Tip 50 - Brain Cells Regrow After All

1. Olaf Bergmann, Kirsty L. Spalding, and Jonas Frisén. Adult Neurogenesis in Humans. Cold Spring Harbor Perspectives in Biology. 2015.

2. Kirsty L. Spalding, Olaf Bergmann, Kanar Alkass, et al. Dynamics of hippocampal neurogenesis in adult humans. Cell. 2013.

3. Pasko Rakic. Discovering the Brain. The Development and Shaping of the Brain. National Academy of Sciences. 1992.

4. Brain Basics: The Life and Death of a Neuron. NIH National Institute of Neurological Disorders and Stroke (NINDS).

5. P S Eriksson, E Perfilieva, T Björk-Eriksson, A M Alborn, C Nordborg, D A Peterson, F H Gage. Neurogenesis in the adult human hippocampus. Nature Medicine. 1998.

6. Elizabeth Gould, Alison J. Reeves, Michael S. A. Graziano, Charles G. Gross. Neurogenesis in the Neocortex of Adult Primates. Science. 1999.

7. Maura Boldrini, Camille A. Fulmore, Alexandria N. Tartt, et al. Human Hippocampal Neurogenesis Persists throughout Aging. Cell Stem Cell. 2018.

8. Elena P Moreno-Jiménez, Miguel Flor-García, Julia Terreros-Roncal, et al. Adult hippocampal neurogenesis is abundant in neurologically healthy subjects and drops sharply in patients with Alzheimer's disease. Nature Medicine. 2019.

9. Jon Gil-Ranedo, Eleanor Gonzaga, Karolina J Jaworek, et al. STRIPAK Members Orchestrate Hippo and Insulin Receptor Signaling to Promote Neural Stem Cell Reactivation. Cell Reports. 2019.

10. Xinyu Zhao and Darcie Moore. Neural stem cells: developmental mechanisms and disease modeling. Cell Tissue Research. 2018.

11. Freya Kamel and Jane A. Hoppin. Association of Pesticide Exposure with Neurologic Dysfunction and Disease. Environmental Health Perspectives. 2004.

12. Hao Wang, Megumi T Matsushita. Heavy metals and adult neurogenesis. Current Opinion in Toxicology. 2021.

13. Konstantinos Kagias, Camilla Nehammer, and Roger Pocock. Neuronal Responses to Physiological Stress. Frontiers in Genetics. 2012.

14. Hyo Jung Kang, Bhavya Voleti, Tibor Hajszan, et al. Decreased expression of synapse-related genes and loss of synapses in major depressive disorder. Nature Medicine. 2012.

15. Eberhard Fuchs, PhD and Gabriele Flügge, PhD. Cellular consequences of stress and depression. Dialogues in Clinical Neuroscience. 2004.

16. G B Jensen, B Pakkenberg. Do alcoholics drink their neurons away? The Lancet. 1993.

17. Debora Melo Van Lent, Hannah Gokingco, Meghan I. Short, et al. Higher Dietary Inflammatory Index scores are associated with brain MRI markers of brain aging: Results from the Framingham Heart Study Offspring cohort. Alzheimer's & Dementia. 2022.

18. Pauline H Croll, Trudy Voortman, M Arfan Ikram, et al. Better diet quality relates to larger brain tissue volumes. Neurology. 2018.

19. I. Figueira, G. Garcia, R. C. Pimpão, A. P. Terrasso, et al. Poly-

phenols journey through blood-brain barrier towards neuronal protection. Scientific Reports Nature. 2017.

20. Kirk I Erickson, Michelle W Voss, Ruchika Shaurya Prakash, et al. Exercise training increases size of hippocampus and improves memory. PNAS. 2011.

21. Katharina Wittfeld, Carmen Jochem, Marcus Dörr, et al. Cardiorespiratory Fitness and Gray Matter Volume in the Temporal, Frontal, and Cerebellar Regions in the General Population. Mayo. 2020.

22. Christopher N. Cascio, Matthew Brook O'Donnell, Francis J. Tinney, et al. Self-affirmation activates brain systems associated with self-related processing and reward and is reinforced by future orientation. Social Cognitive and Affective Neuroscience. 2016.

23. Melinda T. Owens and Kimberly D. Tanner. Teaching as Brain Changing: Exploring Connections between Neuroscience and Innovative Teaching. The American Society for Cell Biology. 2017.

www.ingramcontent.com/pod-product-compliance
Lightning Source LLC
Chambersburg PA
CBHW060453030426
42337CB00015B/1570